PRAISE FOR INTELLIGENT YOGA

'I consider Peter to be one of the most high-integrity leaders of a major par
conceive of, and therefore how we exist within and relate to, the human body.
dogma under the bus, always willing to let his inquiry deepen and expand, this book is a gift to those
who are engaging with their bodies as a lived experience or who are helping others
to do so; whether yoga teachers, movement educators, or bodyworkers of any stripe.'
Brooke Thomas, Liberated Body podcast

'Peter Blackaby's aptly named Intelligent Yoga is a true game-changer for anyone
willing to ask the tough questions of how and why we do yoga. I highly recommend it
to all my serious students.'
Leslie Kaminoff, co-author of *Yoga Anatomy*

'Peter Blackaby's writing (like his teaching) is intelligent, incisive, gracious and immensely pragmatic.
He is proposing shifts in our assumptions about anatomy, asana and teaching that are much
needed – in yoga, and in any movement practice. I highly recommend that everyone engage with
the ideas in this book.'
Amy Matthews, co-author of *Yoga Anatomy*

'Peter Blackaby has a rare gift for expressing his deeply felt understanding for yoga through the written word.
This book captures the essence of his enquiring nature while providing a distinctive method and practice
suggestions which might equally serve the total beginner and the seasoned practitioner. Substantially revised
and updated from the first edition, it is humane, rigorous and refreshing in equal measure. The illustrations
exhibit the very qualities of light, spacious stability and ease that the practice evokes. By the simple device of
stating a purpose (rather than a list of supposed benefits), a method and a sense of enquiry in each asana,
he initiates the intelligent approach that characterises his teaching. This is what I love about his work.
Any body of any shape or size can take this approach and find freedom to move optimally with ease
and grace. It really is essential reading for every modern yoga practitioner.'
Tara Fraser, author of *Yoga for You* and the *The Easy Yoga Workbook*

'Yoga is undergoing a massive paradigm shift. People in the West have been practising yoga for long
enough to start questioning some of the things that the gurus taught. People have gotten injured from
yoga practice and had to explore other modalities and information to heal. Fortunately, Peter Blackaby
is at the forefront of a fantastic new conversation around synthesising knowledge and evolving yoga
practice to incorporate new understandings of how the body works, the role of physical practice in
addressing pain, and larger questions into the nature of being. In his new edition of Intelligent Yoga,
he offers a clear lens that both allows for scientific rigor yet still advocates for the innate wisdom at the
heart of yogic inquiry. Anyone who feels a passion for yoga deserves to read this book.'
J. Brown, yoga teacher, writer, podcaster

'A teacher's plea for safety through individualisation and anatomic savvy.' (first edition)
William J. Broad, author of *The Science of Yoga: The Risks and the Rewards*

'I have been a yoga practitioner for 20 years and teaching for 12 years. I have over 100 books on yoga
but I turn to this one for inspiration more often than any other. I cannot recommend it highly enough.'
(first edition)
Sally A. Furness, on Amazon UK

INTELLIGENT
YOGA

LISTENING TO THE BODY'S INNATE WISDOM

PETER BLACKABY

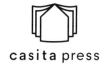

casita press

INTELLIGENT
YOGA

LISTENING TO THE BODY'S INNATE WISDOM

PETER BLACKABY

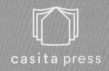

casita press

Published by Casita Press in 2018

ISBN 978-1-5272-2115-4

Author
Peter Blackaby

Publisher, Editor & Production
Anna Norman

Art Director
Samuel Blagg

Proofreaders
Ros Sales and Richard Norman

Indexer
Ros Sales

Photographer
Charlotte Macpherson
(www.charlottemacpherson.co.uk)

Additional photography
p.15 istock.com/SolStock; p.16 Alena Vezza/Shutterstock.com; p.19 franco lucato/Shutterstock.com;
p.27 istock.com/FatCamera; p.28 Institute of Oriental Studies, St. Petersburg, Russia/Bridgeman
Images; p.31 fizkes/Shutterstock.com; p.33 Pan Xunbin/Shutterstock.com; p.34 Pete Saloutos/
Shutterstock.com; p.35 JonathanC Photography/Shutterstock.com; p.37 istock.com/Imgorthand;
p.42 Ivanko80/Shutterstock.com; p.43 lolloj/Shutterstock.com; p.45 Popperfoto/Getty Images;
p.46 Inu/Shutterstock.com; p.49 AYakovlev/Shutterstock.com and istock.com/bauhaus1000; p.50
Henny Allis/Science Photo Library; p.51 imageBROKER/Alamy Stock Photo; p.54 Christine
Hanscomb/Science Photo Library; p.56 Cultura/Science Photo Library; p.64 fizkes/Shutterstock.com;
p.70 Supavadee butradee/Shutterstock.com; p.71 Wellcome Collection. CC BY; p.72 istock.com/
RobertCrum; p.74 Tyler Olson/Shutterstock.com; p.75 Astrakan Images/Getty Images; p.76 Kenny
Tong/Shutterstock.com; p.77 Shaiith/Shutterstock.com; p.81 Edvard Munch/Dag Fosse/KODE;
p.82 Martchan/Shutterstock.com; p.85 Daxiao Productions/Shutterstock.com; p.86 eye-blink/
Shutterstock.com; p.89 Pablo Picasso/Detroit Institute of Arts, USA/Bequest of Robert H. Tannahill/
Bridgeman Images; p.90 Helen Hotson/Shutterstock.com; p.91 Standret/Shutterstock.com; p.185
Don Pablo/Shutterstock.com; p.187 Ilya Andriyanov/Shutterstock.com

Illustrations on pages 60, 63 and 65 by Nicola Fee

The second edition of this book is published in the United Kingdom in 2018 by Casita
Press. Casita Press, The Print House, 18-22 Ashwin Street, London, E8 3DL, UK.

Printed and bound by Gutenberg Press Ltd., Tarxien, GXQ 2901, Malta,
www.gutenberg.com.mt.

The first edition of this book was published in the United Kingdom in 2012 by
Outhouse Publishing, Brighton.

Acknowledgements
The author would particularly like to thank the following for help in shaping this book:
Christine McHugh, Diane Farrell, Taravajra, Peter Connolly and Lisa McRory, for their
generous sharing of ideas and practice – I value their friendship; Mary Stewart for her
straightforward and direct teaching; Serge Gracovetsky for his patient answering of
my persistent questions; Monica Voss for her conversation and encouragement; and
Michael Barnes for introducing me to the wonderful world of yoga. Finally, thanks to
my wife Sabine, and Dominik, my son, who have had to put up with me when my
time has been consumed by writing. The author and editor would also like to thank the
following for modelling the asanas so patiently for us: Mia Dafe, Christine McHugh,
Lisa McRory, Anil Rawal, Taravajra and Ann Thomson.

This book is available from selected bookshops and online booksellers. You can
alternatively buy it directly from Peter Blackaby's website: www.intelligentyoga.co.uk.

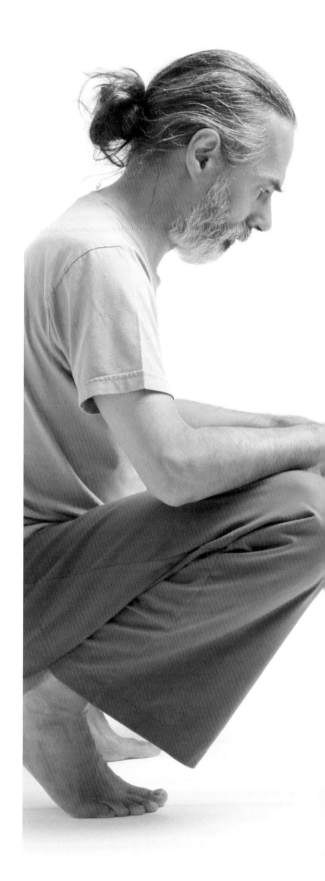

CONTENTS

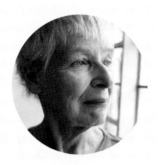

— MARY STEWART —

FOREWORD TO THE FIRST EDITION

Yoga is India's gift to the world. Pre-dating both Hinduism and Buddhism, it was handed down verbally from teacher to pupil for hundreds of years before it was ever committed to paper.

Most people in the West have heard of yoga, perhaps as a form of keep-fit practised by celebrities, as a weekly class in a local village hall, or even as a dangerous Eastern cult. Yoga has been interpreted in innumerable ways over its long history and there is probably a grain of truth in all its many descriptions.

> **'As yoga transforms our relationship with our physical selves, our ability to release effort and let go will bring self-knowledge.'**

Yoga as the path to 'wholeness' has been taught, elaborated, elucidated, muddled, mystified, hidden and even patented. The huge surge of interest in yoga practice in the West over the past forty or so years has only added to the confusion, and modern marketing methods continue to spread images of chanting and extreme exercise routines in which the essentials of yoga practice are all too often lost.

The Sanskrit word 'yoga' means concentration, but it can also be translated as union. Yoga is additionally defined as 'the stilling of the restless state of the mind.' The ancient yoga aphorisms of Patanjali advocate an eight-fold path to this end state, the first two steps of which are ethical and moral rules. The third and fourth steps concern bodily posture and the regulation of the breath, and it is these steps, themselves a preparation for the later steps of meditation, which are mostly taught and practised in the West today.

Yoga, being extremely old, has little in common with modern aerobic exercise routines and physical training, despite attempts to market it thus.

'Postures should be steady and relaxed,' state the aphorisms. They should be performed by releasing and letting go rather than the through use of effort or force. The postures are a concentration of mind and movement in which the breath undoes the stiffness and tensions of the body, strengthening its weaknesses and restoring health.

As yoga transforms our relationship with our physical selves, our ability to release effort and let go will bring self-knowledge. Doing so is as difficult for the young and flexible as it is for those of us who are older and stiffer.

A sound understanding of our physical selves is essential to those students and teachers wishing to embark on their own yoga journey, and this is what Peter provides here, on the pages of *Intelligent Yoga*.

Mary Stewart
London, May 2012

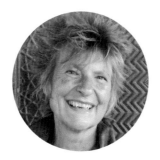

—— MONICA VOSS ——

FOREWORD TO THE SECOND EDITION

The version of yoga presented here promotes optimum health through increased awareness. The concepts have been developed through experimentation and logic; feeling and movement are beautifully integrated. Pete relies on a commonsense, methodical, even-tempered, holistic approach that contributes to recovering ideal movement – variable, soft and pliant, energised, yet never forced or extreme – and, as an important byproduct, this process settles the mind.

Pete expresses his knowledge of anatomy simply and generously. He has studied widely and can explain physiology, neurology, developmental stages, evolution and even delves into anthropology. He's an explorer and an examiner and his landscape and environment are the body and mind. As a result, his work is both intellectually interesting and completely applicable to daily activity.

But more than that, the ideas you'll discover in this book will encourage existential reflection on how we interact in our world and how we want to spend our time, our intelligence and our talents. How do we want to live our lives?

Pete's message can be profound and will motivate many people to analyse and ponder their physical response to the world. 'Normal', he says, is what we do, day-to-day unconsciously, but 'natural' is something else. Naturalness in movement includes freedom of expression, smooth and graceful transitions, easy breathing and confident grounding. These qualities can be rediscovered with precise attention, patience, repetition and self-enquiry, supported by an empathetic instructor and eventually on our own. We learn gradually to clarify for ourselves what's happening now, what's not and what could be.

Yoga is deeply interested in the conservation of energy. If we spend only the energy that is required, we'll have surplus to devote to endeavours that uplift and reward. If yoga teaches us to save energy and is in itself satisfying, we're doubly supported. Pete's yoga practice seems to do just that.

> 'We learn gradually to clarify for ourselves what's happening now, what's not and what could be.'

Intelligent Yoga espouses using quiet attention, thoughtful observation and careful undoing of tension so that what is unnecessary can drop away and dissolve each time we practise. With Pete's approach, we can recoup, rediscover, evolve, learn something new, remember something important. We might recover past abilities; we can experience pleasure in the present and create lasting positive change. All of us, no matter our age, gender, state of being or level of experience, can learn, from Pete's techniques, how to release encumbrances and regain ease, grace and comfort as we move through our world.

Monica Voss
Toronto, February 2018

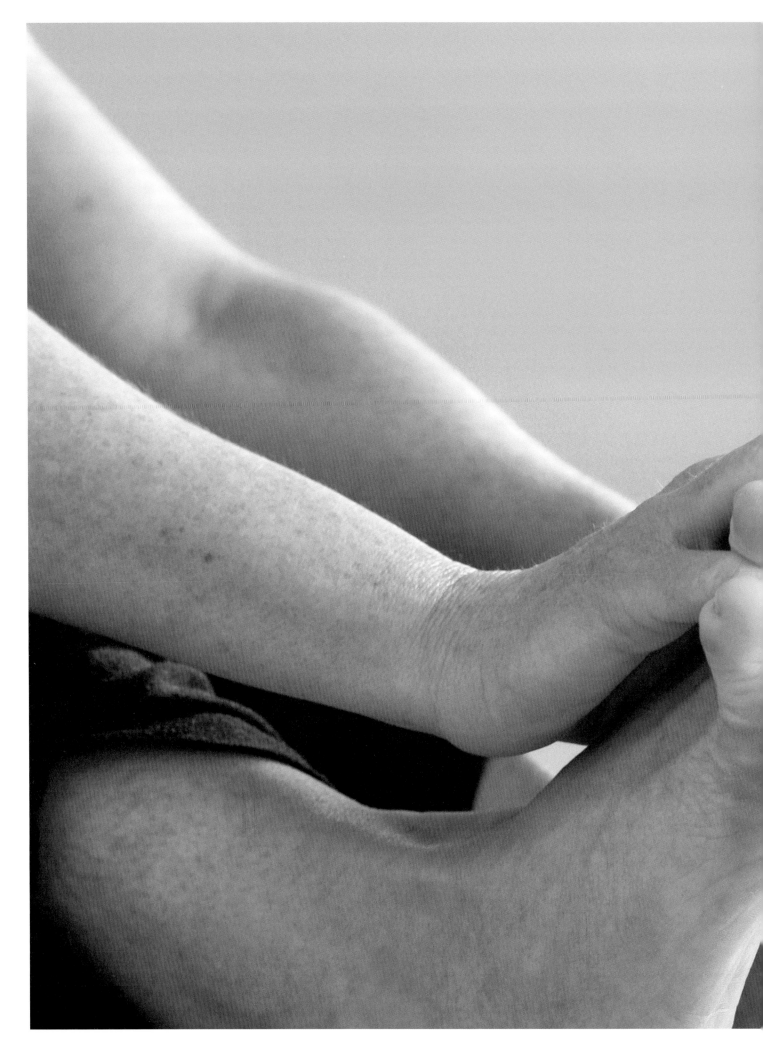

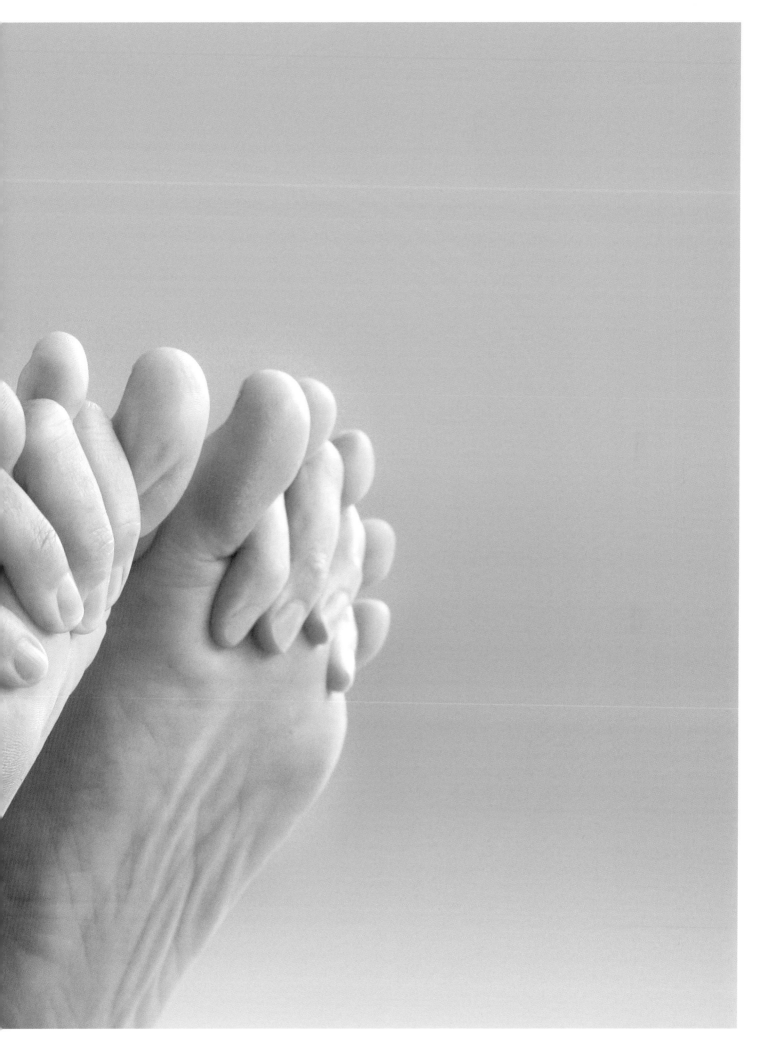

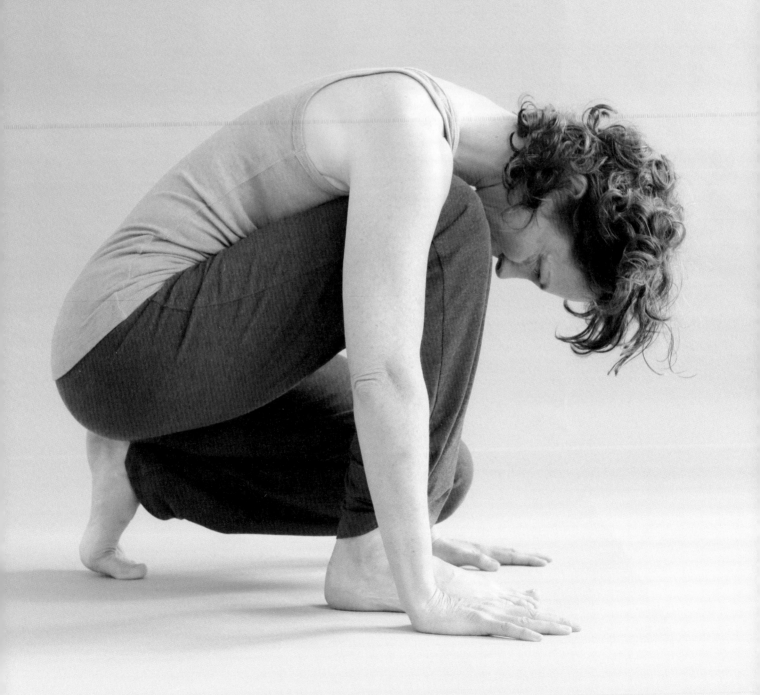

COMING TO OUR SENSES

An intention-based approach to yoga

When I set out to write the first edition of *Intelligent Yoga* there were two main themes in my mind. One was to try to reframe yoga in a modern Western context, shorn of Hindu cultural notions, and the other to argue that there was still something profound in the investigation of the human condition using the body as the entry point. I wanted to show how by approaching yoga from the perspective of Western humanistic psychology and philosophy we can keep the discipline as alive and relevant as possible. The second theme overlapped with the first: to argue that modern yoga practice has followed uncritically the physical teachings of a few leading Indian gurus, and that it was time to review and critique these teachings in the light of modern anatomical and biomechanical understandings, and change them when they were found wanting. It seems that our uncritical acceptance of the vertical transmission of knowledge from guru to student closed our eyes to some ideas that would have been challenged if put forward by Western teachers of exercise and movement. It is perhaps ironic that much of what was being taught in the second half of the twentieth century by people like B.K.S. Iyengar, K. Pattabhi Jois and T.K.V. Desikachar – considered the godfathers of mainstream yoga practice today – was a mishmash of Western and Indian ideas, a theme explored in some depth by both James Mallinson

(*Roots of Yoga*) and Mark Singleton (*Yoga Body*).

This second edition of my book came about because my thinking has evolved – in line with changing ideas about the way the body/self is organised – since the first book was written five years ago. And also because our understanding of the way pain and discomfort arise has also developed since the first edition. I feel no conflict with the first edition, however; rather, I see this edition as reflecting my thought processes – which inevitably move on and develop over time. I hope that many readers will find the revised book a useful stepping-stone in their own journey towards understanding the complexities that make us human.

WHOLE BODY MOVEMENTS

So, which elements of the book have changed the most since the first edition? The main changes are twofold. The first major development stems from my deepening recognition that no living thing exists in isolation. This is true whether we think of a cell existing within the tissues and organs of the body, or whether we think of communities of people living in their environment on the planet. Wherever we look, we see that the health and survival of living things are dependent on the system within which they are embedded, and that the health of the system is of paramount importance if the organism is going to thrive.

It is true that yoga has historically often posited an integrative view of existence. However, though many teachers pay lip service to a holistic approach, in reality the concept has to some extent been lost in modern yoga practice – and particularly in asana work. Reintroducing the concept has several implications when it comes to teaching or practising asana. It means that when we look at the impact of movement on a human being, we need to take into account how *freely* a person moves, how *much* of a person is involved in the movement, how it makes the person *feel*, and also whether the yoga class as a group feels comfortable and safe. These are the sorts of considerations that move to the front of my thinking when I teach. These days, I very rarely think about a 'bit' of a person. For example, I wouldn't teach a class for 'hamstrings', 'the core', 'hip joints' or any other part of the body; I think this is a mistake in thinking. When we think in terms of parts of the body, we can fall into something called the 'mereological fallacy', a concept used to describe the tendency to ascribe to a part of a thing the quality of the whole. In living things, solutions are rarely found in a part, because the part has no meaning when looked at alone – it only has meaning when considered as part of the whole. Solutions are usually found in the *relationship* between parts. So in

> 'Bottom-up processing describes the way an organism responds to its environment through its senses.'
>
> ———

yoga, if someone has a knee problem, it is not usually helpful to focus on the knee, but it might be very helpful to look at the relationship between the knee and the rest of the body as the person moves.

This way of looking at things has moved me further away still from the Western reductionist view of anatomy – where we learn about origins and insertions, agonists and antagonists – towards a view where we think more about the *intention* of a movement, and then about whether a body is compliant with that intention. In other words, does the whole body become involved in the efficient carrying out of a task? And if not, how can we improve the response of the person to the task?

BOTTOM-UP PROCESSING

The second theme that has developed since the first edition is a more consolidated move towards 'bottom-up processing' – as opposed to 'top-down processing'. Bottom-up processing describes the way an organism responds to its environment through its senses. In its simplest form it is drinking water when you are thirsty, resting when you are tired or laughing when you are happy. To do these simple things you first have to notice how you feel; then you have to act appropriately on your feelings in order to feel comfortable again. It is related to the previous argument in that for living things to be connected through systems, there must be a method of connection – a way that we can engage with our environment. In human beings this method of connection happens via our nervous systems. (There are molecular forms of communication as well, but these are not perceptible in the same way.) We notice and respond to our environment through our sensory nervous system and what we notice is then acted on through our muscular system. How well we can respond is clearly going to be related to how accurately we notice things, and this is where yoga practice remains such a useful tool.

We can think of the sensory nervous system as having two main aspects. One aspect concerns the five senses that are most familiar to us, and that help us engage with the world – sight, sound, hearing, smell and touch, with a sixth less obvious one being proprioception, the sense of the relative position of one's body in space and movement. The other aspect of the sensory nervous system is concerned with interoception, or the way we notice the *internal* state of our body. This may be an awareness of anxiety through faster breathing, a change in body temperature and a faster heart rate, or a sense of relaxation because the opposite has occurred.

The whole point of the sensory nervous system is to inform us how we need to modify behaviour to maintain homeostasis.

How we *process* what we notice will be modified by past experiences and sometimes distorted unhelpfully. For instance, after the terrible events of 9/11, some people who had watched the events in New York City unfold in front of them later found themselves suffering from what came to be termed 'blue sky anxiety'. The catastrophe of the two planes flying into the Twin Towers happened against a clear blue backdrop, and some people's minds then started to subconsciously associate clear blue skies with danger.

Whilst it may have been helpful for our primitive ancestors to have clear associations between places and danger, in the modern world this is less often the case, and we can find ourselves triggered into inappropriate responses to particular stimuli by previous association. When this happens we need to re-notice our feeling states and slowly learn to dissociate them from any triggering circumstance.

'The whole point of the sensory nervous system is to inform us how we need to modify behaviour to maintain homeostasis.'

BELOW
Responding to thirst by drinking water is a simple example of bottom-up processing.

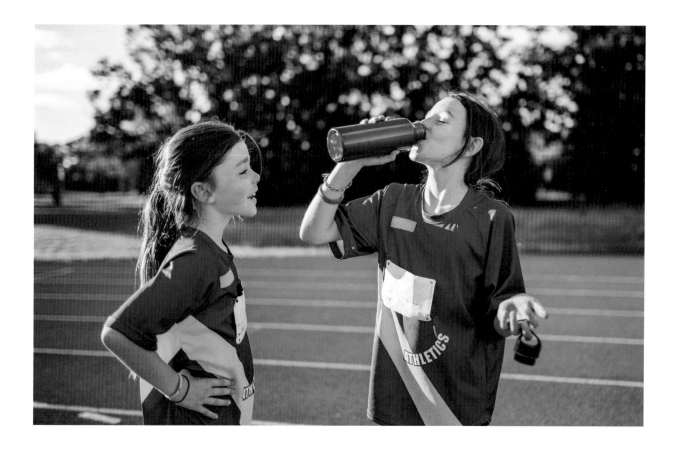

15

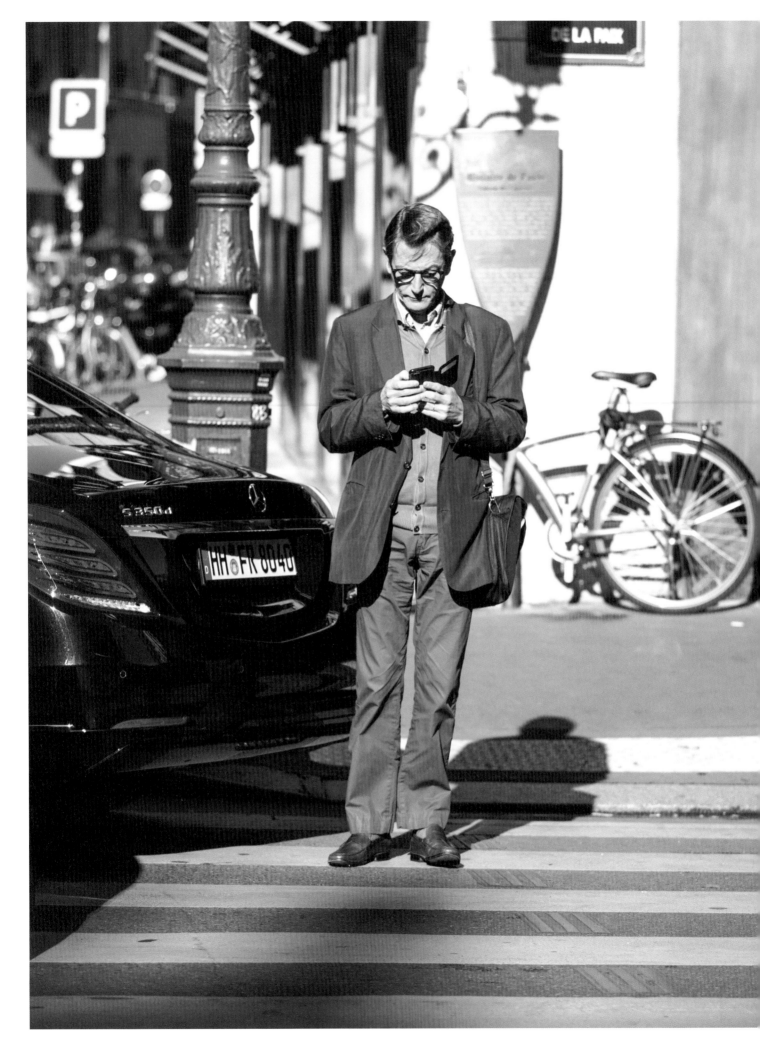

LOSING OUR SENSES

Modern living has muted our ability to sense things well. Our nervous system evolved under evolutionary pressure and our hunter-gatherer ancestors will have honed their senses in life or death situations; their footsteps would have often had to be silent, their movements fluid so as not to attract attention, and their hearing perfectly attuned to their surroundings. In the modern world, on the other hand, we walk on flat, safe surfaces; our movements can be clumsy, at no real cost to our survival; and we have no need to hone our senses, as we are 'kept safe' by any number of warning signs – beeping sounds, hand-rails and announcements telling us to 'mind the gap'! (Experiments concerned with reversing this societal trend have been undertaken. The Dutch road traffic engineer Hans Monderman pioneered the idea of doing away with traffic lights and other road markings, to see if drivers then pay more attention. Accident rates plummeted.) It seems that this 'muting' of our sensory signals in our modern world leads to a gradual confusion of how we actually feel in ourselves, resulting in odd migrating pains in our muscles and joints, recurring headaches and digestive ailments, and psychological feelings of disquiet, anxiety or depression.

There is another way we become disconnected from our bodies, which has attracted a lot of attention in the last decade, and that is through emotional trauma. If something deeply shocking happens to us, we tend to shut down the part of the brain that helps us make sense of internal feelings. In effect, we try to hide from our feelings. Although this may be useful in the short term, because those feelings may threaten to overwhelm us, in the long term it means we become unable to interpret our 'gut feelings' accurately. In such cases we can easily overreact to stimuli, and develop panic attacks or other disturbing bodily symptoms in response to

LEFT
Modern technology, such as traffic lights and mobile phones, mute our ability to develop sensory awareness.

apparently innocuous events. We will look at this in more detail in chapter three, but it is worth mentioning here that many people are now arguing that somatic intervention into psychological and physical trauma is deeply effective. Amongst the leading lights in this field are Bessel Van Der Kolk, Stephen Porges, Peter Lavine and Stanley Keleman, all of whom have contributed enormously to the field of trauma therapy.

LEARNING TO RE-NOTICE

So how do we reconnect ourselves if we have become fragmented by life? I would certainly put my weight behind the perspective that we have in one way or another to learn to re-notice ourselves. And yoga is extremely well placed to facilitate this, particularly if it means paying attention to things we have previously left unacknowledged and that we take for granted – the sensations we have when we practise. This might mean noticing the feeling of muscles stiffening as they take up the work of a posture, then releasing and softening again as the work subsides. It might be the feeling of contact with the floor through a foot or hand, or any other body part that is in contact with the ground. Other things we can notice are the fluidity of a movement, the acceleration and deceleration of the body in transition from one place to another, the sense of weight through bones, and the feeling of spaciousness or constriction in the chambers of the body. In our yoga practice we are to some extent trying to pay attention to ourselves in the way our ancient ancestors might have had to in order to survive. Moving through the jungle or the savannah in a way that does not draw attention to oneself requires a particular sense of embodiment and care in quiet, smooth movement. There is an alertness and presence apparent, but not the type of frowning concentration often present in modern life.

This approach to yoga, a 'bottom-up approach', is a marked shift away from the 'exercise' approach, peppered with basic Eastern philosophy, so popular in mainstream modern yoga practice. It has more in common with other Western systems like the Alexander Technique, the Feldenkrais Method,

'What I am interested in is working with the nervous system. It is increasingly apparent that it is here that most of our problems and, conversely, solutions lie.'

People from hunter-gatherer societies often have a greater sensory connection to their surroundings.

Somatics and Body-Mind Centering. I am no longer interested in the focus on structure, and on stretching and strengthening the muscles and fascia of the body. Of course, if you work with the body, it will change: muscles will become stronger and range of movement will improve if these things are needed – but only if the function demands it. Lengthening and strengthening are not the aim, they are the side effects of practice. What I am interested in is working with the nervous system, because it is becoming increasingly apparent that it is here that most of our problems and, conversely, solutions lie. This approach to yoga also encompasses a more serious attempt to integrate us as human beings, firstly with ourselves, the body/mind; then with our fellow humans; and finally with the greater world outside. This book approaches this subject as follows.

In **chapter one**, I will take issue with the reductionist/structuralist model that still seems so prevalent in modern yoga practice, and identify how it has come about and why it has so often gone unchallenged. Unfortunately, one of the main places that this model has become entrenched is in yoga teacher training programmes, where the emphasis still seems to be on the origin, insertion and function of particular muscles, and where students are encouraged to focus on which muscles are involved in which asanas. The problem with this way of thinking is that if a student cannot perform an asana they will tend to look for the 'bit/muscle' that is wrong, and this leads to a misunderstanding of how the body is organised. So in chapter one I want to put forward a more helpful way of approaching asana (i.e. physical yoga practice) that is more in line with the way we are really organised. This focuses on *functional* human movement and how these patterns are organised in the brain, with an emphasis on body compliance, or how much of the body participates in any given movement.

In **chapter two**, I want to argue for a different way of seeing anatomy in relation to movement, which focuses on putting things together rather

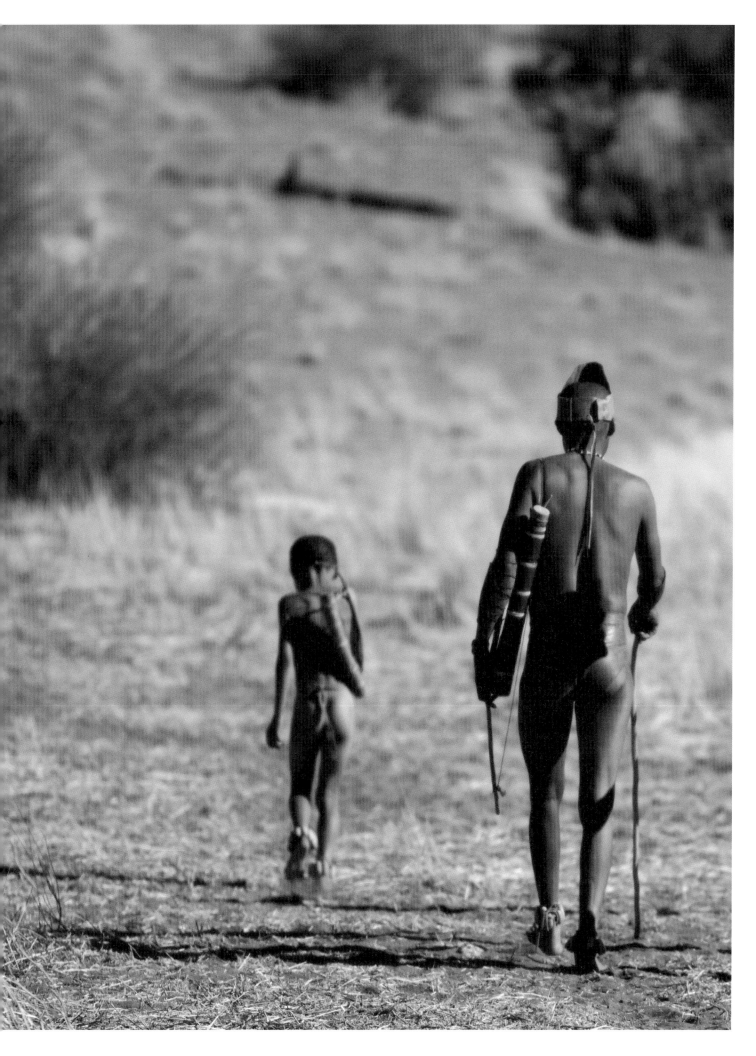

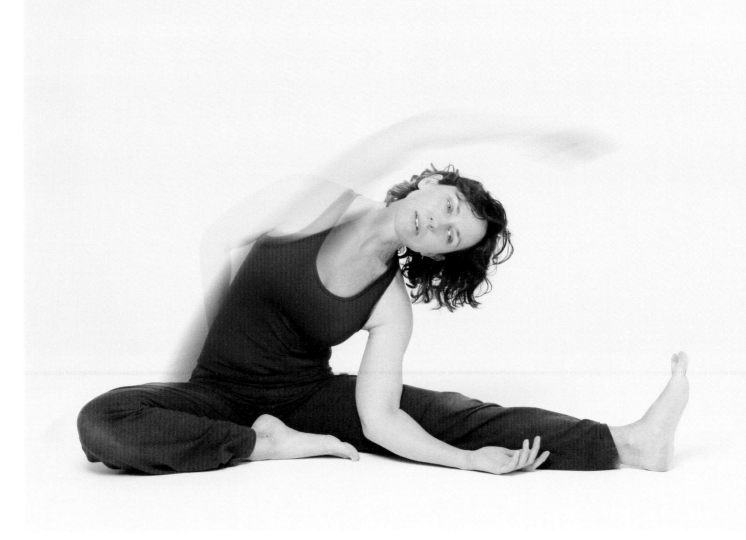

ABOVE
Yoga can help us become more
fully integrated as human beings.

than taking them apart. I particularly want to
emphasise the role of the nervous system in this
process, with attention paid to the way we map
the body in the sensorimotor cortex. We will look
at how muscles respond to support by relaxing,
and how this tends to free up movement. In this
way of looking at asana we see bones as a means
of support, which if used appropriately will reduce
tension in muscles. We will see fascia/connective
tissue as a means of providing tensional support
and distribution of forces across the body, and the
muscles and nervous system coordinating intention

in the most efficient way possible. I also introduce
the idea of compliance and differentiation and
ways of thinking about how to achieve this.

In **chapter three**, I explain how breathing and
postural support influence each other. We need to
move away from the idea that there are postural
muscles, respiratory muscles and functional muscles
as separate categories. All muscles will, when
necessary, be recruited for the task at hand, whether
it be a yoga posture or pulling a weed out of a flower
bed. No muscle is assigned a special task on its own;
instead, muscles are recruited to help carry out the
intention of the person as competently as possible.

This is not the view we get from anatomy
books that describe a bicep as an elbow flexor
or the quadriceps as knee extensors; that view is
misleading and unhelpful. Breathing is a global
event causing shape change in both the upper and

lower chambers of the body. This chapter thus also looks at the relationship between these two chambers and how they influence each other, and in particular how we can free up the breath by using bandhas in our yoga practice. Other aspects related to breathing, such as the health of the organs, are also examined.

'The dance between conforming to our species and culture, and maintaining our individuality, is what keeps our practice alive, fresh and ever-interesting.'

————

In **chapter four**, I address how things can go wrong in the body, leading to pain, and what we can do about it. In the last decade, a great deal of research has moved our understanding of pain and discomfort forward. New paradigms to explain pain have emerged, as have ideas on dealing with trauma. Neuroscientists have mapped the brain more thoroughly and there is growing recognition that the physiological body, with all its sensory input, plays a vital role in the formation of emotions and certain aspects of consciousness. When the body or the emotions become 'disregulated' in life, and we become unwell, how we attend to the feelings we notice in our body can play a major part in our recovery.

If we take these ideas on board it will inevitably change the way we practise and teach yoga. Again, we will find ourselves drawn away from the idea of yoga as an 'exercise system' towards the idea of yoga being a route to help us become fully integrated as human beings.

In **chapter five**, I want to stand back and look at human beings in relationship to the world, finding a thread that joins physiology with psychology and philosophy – not as separate subjects but as a way

of being in the world, a way of being that has at its source the intention of reducing suffering and promoting flourishing. It is also helpful to look at our evolutionary history to see how human beings have become what we are. This helps provide some context to both body and mind and enables us to see what it is that we share with other humans – the things that are common to us all. Then we can reflect on our individual history and see how our lives have shaped us as individuals. The dance between conforming to our species and culture, and maintaining our individuality, is what keeps our practice alive, fresh and ever-interesting.

In the second, practice-focused section of the book, I emphasise the importance of having a clear intention to our practice, and a coherent thread that runs through it. I explain my thoughts on this, and on the particular type of attention required to elicit meaningful change in our behaviour and yoga practice, in **chapter six**. I also discuss the theme of grounding here, showing that muscles are unable to relax unless they are supported by the ground via our skeletal system.

I then practically examine individual asanas, breaking this section down into the following chapters. **Chapter seven** covers what I have termed 'tension-losing asanas'; that is, a group of postures and movements whose primary purpose, from my perspective, is to help us to really differentiate between relaxed, working and tense muscles, to allow us to become more efficient in our movements and to reduce habitually held tension. These asanas have a different focus to the bulk of yoga asanas that I practise, which are based around functional movement, and it is these asanas that are covered in **chapter eight**. As it is a big chapter, I have broken it down into five sections: side bends, extension asanas, flexion asanas, rotation asanas and sitting asanas. That leaves balances, which are covered in **chapter nine**. Finally, in **chapter ten** I describe the breathing techniques Uddiyana Bandha and Kapalabhati, both of which are useful for helping to free up the respiratory system. I end with the classic end-of-class relaxation posture, Savasana.

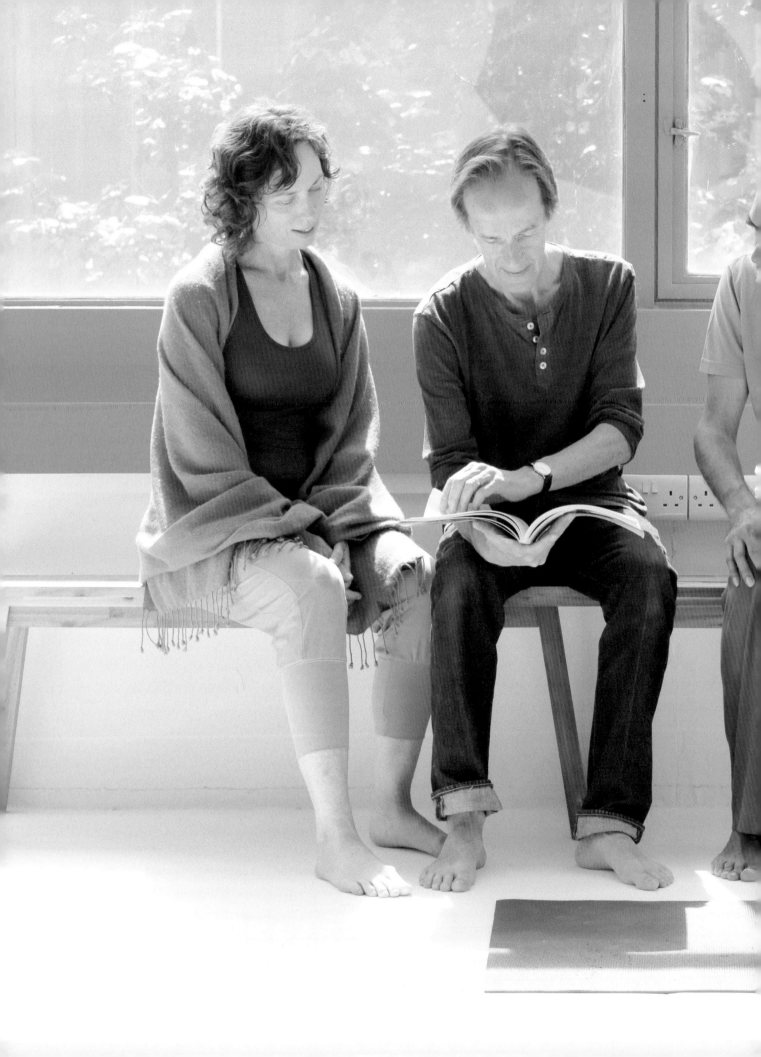

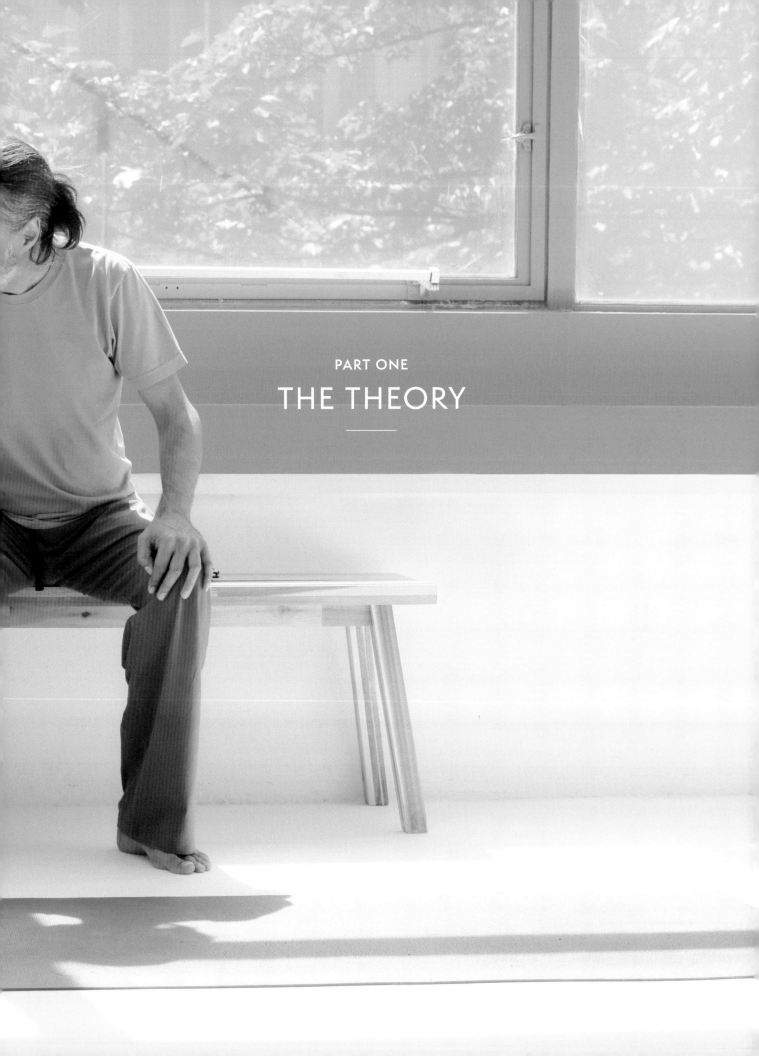

PART ONE
THE THEORY

ONE

FROM SEPARATION
TO INTEGRATION

A functionalist approach to yoga

In the 1960s and '70s, the West fell in love with the East, which seemed to offer answers to questions we in the West had not even asked. The ideas of peace, love and understanding that seemed to permeate Eastern mysticism sat in stark contrast to post-war scientific thinking, with its much-derided Cartesian, reductive approach to life. It seemed that Eastern perspectives offered something richer and deeper than the facile lives being lived in the big cities of the West.

Yoga was part of this movement, and was brought over to the West as something of a cultural package: much of what seemed mysterious and alluring about it was bound to the society and culture in which it was embedded. Ashrams sprang up all over the Western world, while many thousands of people went to India to experience the authentic setting of yoga.

Of course, there were contradictions, and pictures of *sadhus* (holy men) emerging from McDonald's with whopper-sized milkshakes highlighted the ambiguities and complexity of this collision of cultures that we are still shaking down from. When collisions such as this happen, there is an inevitable cross-fertilisation of ideas – some consciously adopted, but others occurring almost by osmosis – and it can take a long time before such ideas

have been sifted enough for sense to be made of them. It has been far too easy to reach ill-informed conclusions about the West or the East, to see these diverse cultures in black and white rather than the many shades of grey that surely exist.

My own journey in both yoga and manual therapy has involved a slow but steady move from a position where I thought people could be 'fixed' by mending their broken parts, towards the view that people do not really 'break'; rather, they gradually move into situations where they do not fit with their bodies as comfortably as they did. And in that uncomfortable place, symptoms – whether physical, psychological, emotional or a mix of the three – are thrown up.

What I have learnt in recent years, however, is that there is no obvious correlation between symptomology and causation. This is in contrast to the view I was taught as an osteopath and Iyengar yoga teacher. In both these disciplines, the approach was a mechanistic one: you looked at the body a little like a machine, examining it for any perceivable engineering issue – a leg that was a little longer on one side, for instance, or an asymmetry of the spine appearing as a scoliosis or kyphosis. These problems could be 'solved' by tightening or strengthening weak, long muscles, and stretching or loosening tight, short muscles, and occasionally

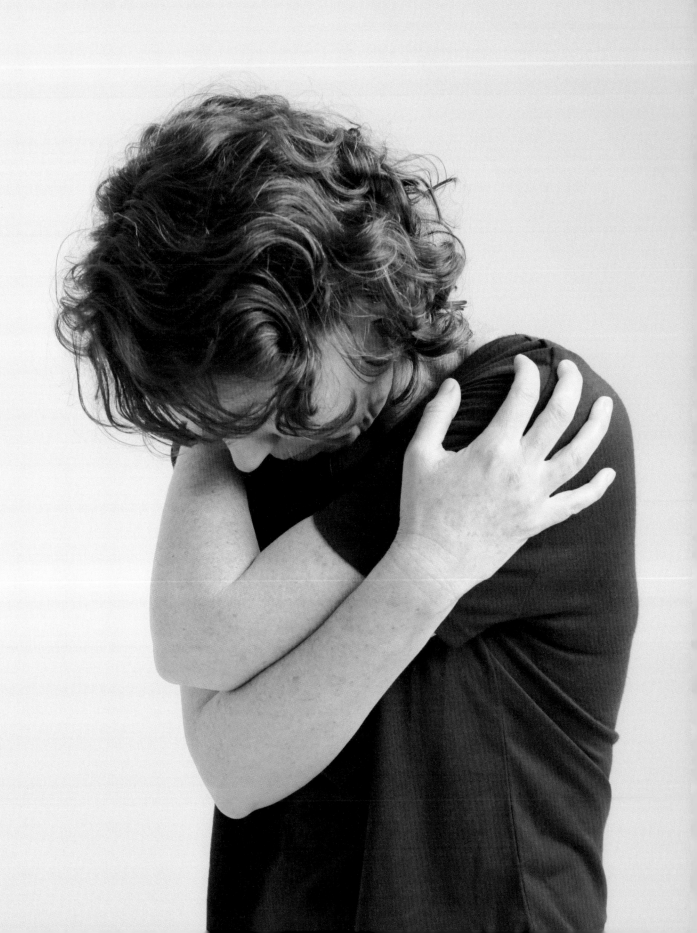

> 'Thinking has become more joined up, and many people have embraced a more holistic, ecological approach.'

_____

pushing a bone back into place. The idea was to pull the frame/skeleton into a better alignment through these adjustments. The body was looked at as something that could be changed by intervening in its structure, as if it was a machine.

I now realise that there are major flaws in this way of thinking. It has become more and more clear to me that bodies are shaped by the way we feel, by the things we do regularly and by conditioned ideas about the way we should look. All of these things are organised at a *neurological* level, not at a structural one, as I shall seek to show in the following chapters. So, my focus of attention has shifted from looking at 'what shape people are in', to asking 'why are people in that shape?' The answers are usually more complex and interwoven than they seemed to be when taking a mechanistic stance... but this reflects the reality of life in general, and my journey has, to some extent, also mirrored the way Western thinking has been changing as a whole.

EVOLVING WESTERN THINKING

The West has been in the middle of some major transformations over the past few decades. Science has led to better understanding of the environment, ecology and the human condition, and thinking is often less reductionist these days; we are starting to better understand the relationship between things. Most people, for example, now realise that not all health problems can be solved by swallowing pills – we know that exercise, diet, stress and environmental factors all play their part in making us healthy or ill. Many now recognise that the initial enthusiasm for the technical fix – in particular through antibiotics and DDT – was scientifically immature. Antibiotics saved millions of

lives when they were first introduced, but an over-reliance on them has led to problems of microbial resistance. Our approach to health has been steadily broadening from a biomedical model, where ill health is treated just by medical means, towards a biopsychosocial model of health, where the psychological and social status of an individual are included in the assessment of wellbeing. Thinking has become more joined up, and many people have embraced a more holistic, ecological approach, while interest in mindfulness meditation has now hit the mainstream. There is, undoubtedly, still a long way to go, but the first steps are being taken.

We have also found flaws in the Indian experience, such as the Bagwan Rajneesh and his Rolls Royces and dubious sexual behavior, and the exposure of Sai Baba as a fraudster and possibly worse (even though excuses are still made for him by his devotees). The iniquities of the caste system and the historical support found for it in some of India's theology and religious texts leave a rather bitter taste in the mouth. We have become more nuanced in our approach, stripping away the culturally specific aspects of yoga that might not be useful or relevant to us and shifting focus to a more systems-based/neurological perspective.

If we reframe yoga, however, and substitute metaphysical ideas with more concrete, naturalistic ones, can we still call it yoga? I believe that there is no loss of dignity in this approach – and that in fact there is a great 'reasonableness' at the centre of yoga that can also be understood in the context of Western culture and science. There are scientific explanations for some of the phenomena that yoga practice brings. The more we are able to use this insight, the greater will be our capacity to adapt and improve what we already have. If yoga is going to continue developing in the West, it is necessary to take it forward within the context of the current Western mind.

THE LANGUAGE OF YOGA

Yoga is largely an experiential practice and its benefits are sometimes difficult to fully articulate. Of course, it is reasonably easy to explain that an

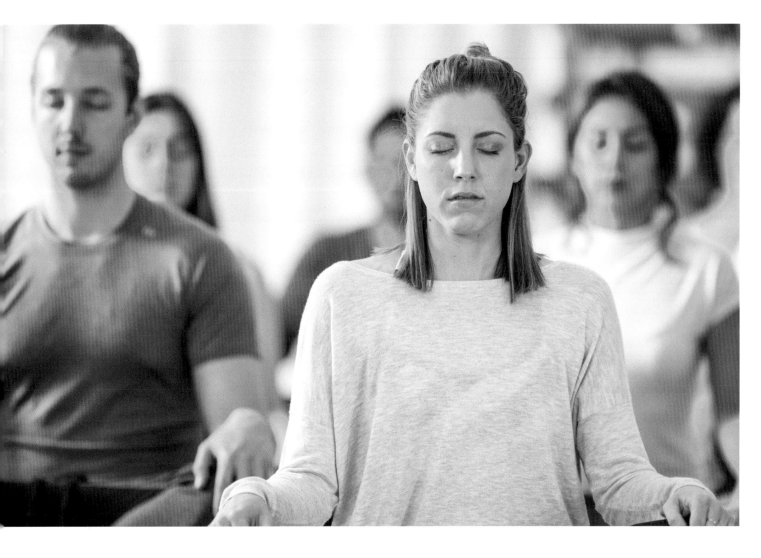

ache or pain has disappeared. What is trickier to explain is the feeling of spaciousness in the body, or the clarity of mind that many people associate with yoga. These things are harder to express and may necessitate the use of imagery or metaphors. Sometimes this is straightforward: the feeling of heaviness or lightness in the body, for example, is something most of us can understand. But how does one speak about the transmission of weight through the bones or the subtle changes in tension we feel in our bodies as we breathe?

If a teacher wishes to convey to students a sensation as clearly as possible, then his or her language will by necessity become increasingly elaborate or subtle. This is where an unquestioning focus on yoga's Eastern heritage can obfuscate things, and where complex culture-specific imagery can lead to misinterpretation. A case in point is the concept of *prana* – the Sanskrit word for the vital life force. If I am on all fours and I pay attention to my body as I exhale, I can feel a sense of weight

ABOVE
Mindfulness meditation has gone from a fringe activity to a mainstream practice.

moving down my arms into the floor. What I am actually feeling is the release of tension that this inhalation necessarily brings into the respiratory system, and the transmission of this release through the bones of the body and into the floor.

This can be perceived as feeling as if you are breathing out through your arms and exhaling down into the floor. Some people might also explain this as the experience of *prana* moving down the *nadis* (channels) of the arm as we exhale. Both ways of describing the experience can be useful in helping people interpret what is felt, and of course different images and descriptions will work for different people.

Problems arise, however, when a description of a 'felt sense' is turned into a statement of fact.

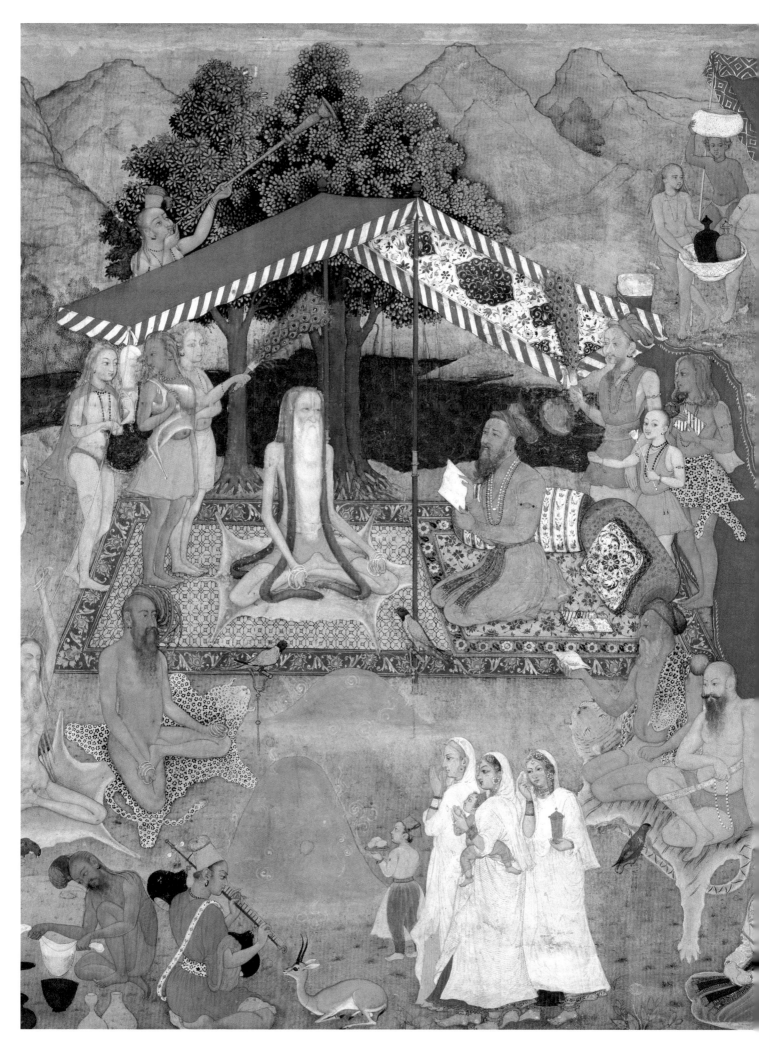

'This nuance in language is based on an important concept: the more powerfully we assert abstract, metaphysical ideas, the less chance we have of allowing people to have their own experience, derived from their own personal practice.'

———

The statement 'It is prana moving down the nadis' brings with it a whole host of assumptions about our physiology, and is quite different to *imagining* it as a possibility. Once an idea becomes concrete it is very difficult to open oneself to another experience, as the mind comes to expect what it has been led to believe. Telling someone what they are feeling is quite different from asking someone to take notice of what they feel.

To discuss yoga practice in any meaningful way we should muster as much clarity as possible. It is all too easy to find oneself donning the emperor's new clothes in an effort to comply with a teacher's wishes. If a student lacks confidence and a teacher suggests that a particular sensation or perception is significant, it is quite likely that the student will say he or she can feel or see what is suggested – whether or not they can. It follows, then, that if we have a naturalistic explanation for a sensation, we should use it. Instead of saying that back bends are good for opening the heart chakra, which I have heard put forward, why not simply explain that they create space in the front of the body? If we do not have a naturalistic explanation, then a neutral image or analogy is better than a quasi-metaphysical one that is difficult for many people to 'get'. This nuance in

LEFT
17th century painting
depicting Indian gurus.

language may seem a small point but it is based on an important concept: the more powerfully we assert abstract, metaphysical ideas, the less chance we have of allowing people to have their own experience, derived from their own personal practice.

A PERSONAL APPROACH
In the early stages, when teaching beginners, yoga classes must be directive to some extent. Students need to understand how to position their bodies in space, and they have to learn the postures, in much the same way as a musician needs to learn the fingering of an instrument. Whereas the goal of the musician is eventually to play music, the goal of the yoga student is to feel comfortable in body, breath and mind, and to integrate these aspects of themselves in such a way that there is little or no conflict between them. Once this happens we can start to become truly healthy.

As well as often being taught yoga through culturally specific language and terms, students are also often encouraged to conform to a particular set of physical and sometimes psychological values. For example, a teacher will provide a sequence of postures to be performed in a particular way, and questioning of any of these postures will be met with an implicit (or sometimes explicit): 'You haven't found the answer because you haven't penetrated the posture deeply enough.' The same can be true when some of the more esoteric ideas in yoga are presented as concrete – for instance, the idea that someone is not experiencing chakras, auras or 'energy' because they are not yet sensitive enough, and that the mystery of these things can be revealed only when you have reached a higher level of understanding.

But what if these things do not actually exist? What if they are phenomena experienced as real by an individual because of his or her personal history and cultural context? Other people may experience them very differently or may never experience them. If this is the case, then any suggestion that these higher states are the result of serious practice can at best only lead to a sense of failure in the student who does not get it, or worse still, lead students away from their own authentic experience towards another, supposedly more desirable one. Being led to conform to a teacher's viewpoint, whatever that viewpoint is, is inevitably disempowering for the student, who becomes dependent on the teacher. This is the opposite of what teaching is supposed to do – which is surely to facilitate learning as effectively as possible.

On top of this over-dependency on the knowledge of the teacher, solutions to problems within the yoga world today are often still sought within the books from ancient India, such as the *Bhagavad Gita*, Patanjali's *Sutras* or the *Upanishads*. Like the Bible in the West, these texts, and others like them, offer useful insights into ways of reducing suffering but, as with the Bible, they are very much of their time and culture, and many aspects of them need serious re-interpretation if they are to make sense nowadays. How much more sensible would it be to regard them as interesting and valuable historical documents, to which have been added a great deal of psychological, philosophical and moral understandings?

Perhaps one of the most challenging aspects of teaching yoga – and indeed of life – is this delicate balance between the needs of the individual and the needs of the community in which we are embedded. A healthy community asks us to surrender some of our autonomy for the good of the group. If we give up too much autonomy, we suffer by not getting our needs met. And if we hold on to too much, the group suffers because of a lack of coherent direction. It is a tricky balancing act to get right. But if a person's experience is to be personal rather than suggested, it is important that this person is quickly allowed to find his own experience, and discover just how it is to inhabit his or her own body. If we start with the individual body, rather than a set of beliefs, then postures can be developed around the body, rather than the body around the postures. And if a problem occurs with a posture or movement, we can look at the posture's 'fit' to the individual and try to improve things. Should a problem arise – 'My knee hurts every time I do this,' for example – one can freely adjust the posture so that it is more compatible with one's individual needs.

THE MECHANICS OF MODERN YOGA POSTURES

It is not only the metaphysical language and guru-led approach we should question, however. Many of the actual asanas practised today should also be critically analysed if we are to clarify what is helpful about yoga.

Modern yoga practice has been shown by authors such as Mark Singleton, Elizabeth De Michelis, N.E. Sjoman and James Mallinson to consist of an eclectic mix of postures, taken from a variety of different sources, including Western gymnastics, body building and Indian wrestling, with some innovations added in. The Indian yoga teacher Tirumalai Krishnamacharya was particularly imaginative in evolving new asanas in the 1920s and '30s, which were further developed by his son T.K.V. Desikachar and student/nephew B.K.S Iyengar in the second half of the twentieth century.

Several of these asanas are problematic, for two main reasons. One is that many of the postures of modern practice have been reduced to being purely a way of stretching or strengthening muscles, as if doing this will be of some long-lasting benefit to the person, when all it really does is enable a person to carry out that particular asana. Kurmasana (Tortoise), Kapotasana (Pigeon) and Hanumanasana (Monkey, or front splits) are good examples of this – postures for which you simply need flexibility to 'perform'. This turns yoga into something more akin to gymnastics than traditional yoga, which is founded on something more than this.

It also makes yoga practice more susceptible to what is known as the 'mereological fallacy'. This describes a way of thinking about things where we wrongly ascribe a value to a part of something that is properly ascribed to the whole. In yoga, this translates into the belief that working on a part of the body will accrue a benefit to the whole. This way of thinking is deeply misleading because movement is actually generated through 'intentions' in the brain and then carried out by the body as an integrated muscular event or sequence, rather than as separated parts – something that I will describe in more detail in chapter two. We slip into this mistake when we think that stretching a hamstring, opening a hip or strengthening the 'core' is an effective way of working on the body. Somewhere in this thinking is the notion that a hamstring has 'become short', a hip has 'become stiff' or the core has 'become weak', as if these areas have an independence from the rest of the human being and have decided to behave in an unhelpful way. This is nonsense. If an area of the body appears tight or weak or stiff, it is generally because of the way a person acts and responds in the world as a whole. If we want to engage with the problems a person presents, we need instead to look at the whole situation, not just where the symptom emerges.

Our thinking needs to centre around how we can help students manage global movements that include their difficult area. The more skilful we are as teachers, the more able we get at inviting a student's 'difficult bit' – their unmapped part – into a useful global movement.

For example, if someone has been identified as having a 'tight iliopsoas', the mechanistic answer would be to stretch it to solve the problem. But this is unlikely to help, because the 'tightness' comes from the way the person moves and notices themselves. A better approach would be to lay someone on their back with their knees bent and feet on the floor, and to then ask them to gently press their feet down. To do this, you employ the muscles that oppose the iliopsoas in their action over the hip, so they are invited to relax. If you then continue to press your feet down, the action will slowly bring the pelvis off the floor but with the iliopsoas relaxed and therefore able to lengthen in the context of a broader movement.

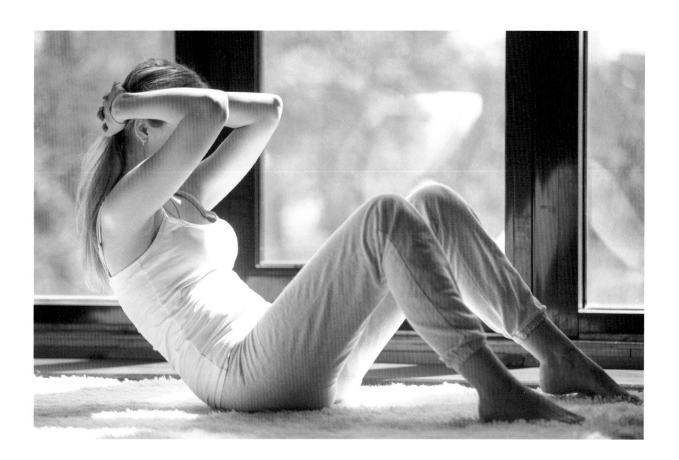

'While anatomy is essential for anyone practising medicine, it is much less useful in helping us to describe movement. After all, every healthy human being learned to move without studying anatomy – as do all animals on the planet.'

I want to make it clear here that I am taking issue with the increasing tendency in yoga, and in yoga teacher training, to focus on bits of the body – particularly individual muscles and joints, and these days also individual types of tissue (namely fascia). These ideas have been imported from the anatomical perspective, and while anatomy is essential for anyone practising medicine, or who might operate on parts of our body, it is much less useful in helping us to describe movement. After all, every healthy human being learned to move without studying anatomy – as do all animals on the planet.

While I have no problem with the desire to study anatomy and physiology – it is a fascinating subject – I do have a problem with the conclusions many anatomists come to regarding movement. There is a tendency to indulge in reverse-engineering, trying to understand movement by looking at the parts rather than understanding that movement starts as an idea/intention in the cortex and is then carried out in the way we have rehearsed such movements throughout our life. If we have not rehearsed a movement well, we need to practise more until we have improved it to our satisfaction. What we should not do is blame the 'bit' that seems tight or weak.

The second problem is that a good number of asanas practised in yoga classes today do not conform well to human anatomy. Very deep back bends, such as King Pigeon (Rajakapotasana), sideways stretching of the spine as found in the Iyengar-style Triangle (Trikonasana), and movements that cause twisting actions in the knee – such as the wide-stride versions of Warrior One (Virabhadrasana I) and Reverse Triangle – can all lead to damage in one way or another, as we will look at in more detail in chapter four. When we decide to move, it makes sense to consider what sorts of movements are most useful to human beings. For the sake of simplicity I will refer to these as 'functional movements'. Deciding which postures are functionally sound for the human body is not easy and opinions here vary. However, I think there are a few things that can guide our ideas about how humans move, and therefore what postures we can practise to support those movements.

FUNCTIONAL MOVEMENT PATTERNS

Our 'guides' for identifying functional movement come from three main sources: scientific research on human evolution, developmental research on how babies have to organise their movements to eventually rise up on to two feet and walk, and ethnographic material that looks at movement from an anthropological perspective across different cultures.

The movements displayed by all mobile life forms have their origins in the pulsations of the invertebrates. The first serious attempts at locomotion developed with muscles acting on a skeleton. In fish, this was through the side-bending movements of the spine, controlled by long lateral and intercostal muscles. When fish left the oceans and pulled themselves on to the land, they evolved into low-slung reptiles, with the legs splayed out to the side. Side-bending was still the preferred method of movement, however; fins eventually became legs, acting at the apex of the side-bending curve and increasing the leverage of side-bending propulsion. The intercostal muscles (the group of muscles between the ribs) in lizards act as both respiratory muscles and locomotor muscles for side-bending.

This is problematic for the lizard, as it means that running and breathing cannot be accomplished at the same time. Running has to be done in short bursts with resting periods in which the lizard can catch its breath.

Serge Gracovetsky, author of *The Spinal Engine*, makes the point that when rotation is brought into the side-bending spine, extension is an inevitable consequence. This is because of something called 'coupled motion of the spine', something that was first observed by American medical doctor R. Lovett in 1905, and backed up by research by orthopaedic surgeons Augustus White and Manohar Panjabi in the 1970s. Back-bending almost certainly developed as a result of the early lizards having to twist their way over obstacles in their path.

In mammals, the diaphragm seems to have evolved with the change in position of the legs. As legs moved from the sides to underneath the body, side-bending became less useful as a means

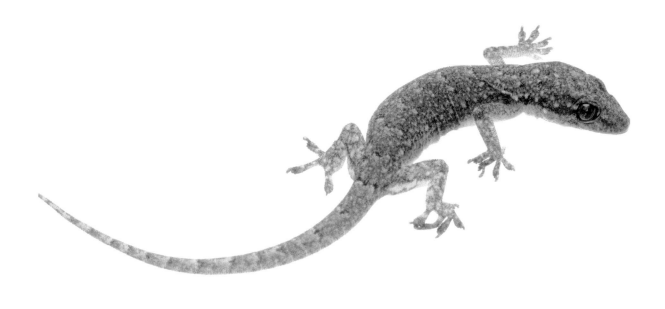

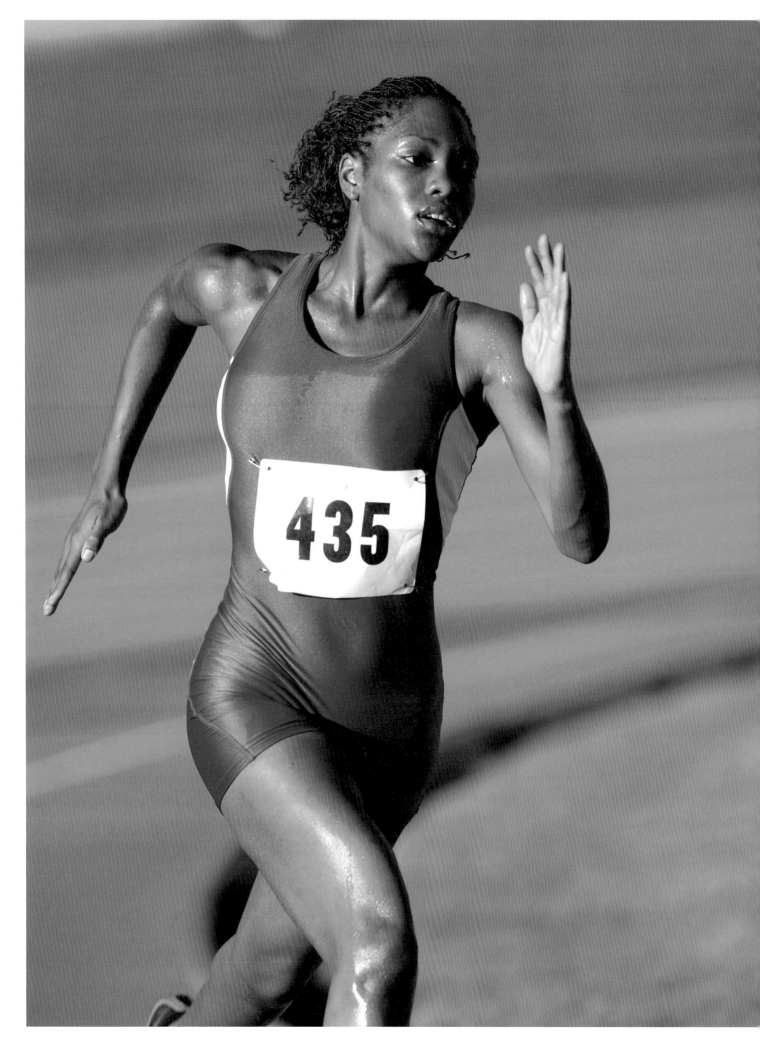

of locomotion, and the ribs remained freer for breathing. Longer legs enabled early mammals to move more easily over objects, and the up and down movements of the spine further developed. The diaphragm and soft belly developed firstly to enable respiration and movement to take place at the same time, and secondly to allow greater flexion and extension of the body – something necessary for swift movement on land. Think of the running cheetah, how its body folds as its feet move together, and extends as the legs reach away from each other. Finally, in human locomotion, rotation forms a fundamental part of our gait – or at least it did with our hunter-gatherer ancestors and still does in the case of modern-day athletes. If we look at shoulder and pelvic movements in Olympic runners, we can see how significant the rotation and counter-rotation movements are.

If we look back over our evolutionary history, we see that our spine has been used to repeatedly side-bend, flex, extend and rotate as part of locomotion, and that although the dominant movements change depending on the type of locomotion being used, the spine has developed a resilience to these movements, and the nervous system an understanding of them. In other words, our bodies can safely reflect these movements, as long as they are not taken to extremes. So it is fairly safe to say that a certain amount of side-bending, flexion, extension and rotation can form a basis for safe and useful yoga practice. If we are teaching movements that do not reflect these patterns, we need to ask ourselves *why* we are teaching them.

In a similar way, we can look at developmental studies to tell us what movements babies go through to establish adult locomotion. As babies grow and develop we notice a generalised pattern of movement behaviours. For a child to make the bridge between being a helpless baby and a free-roaming toddler, the body needs to organise itself in particular ways – ways that are reminiscent of our evolutionary heritage. Side-bending, back-bending, forward-bending and turning movements can all be observed in babies. Although each particular baby may start these movements at a slightly different age, nearly all

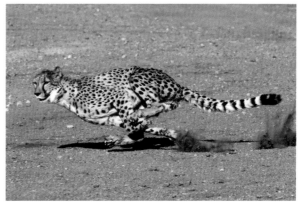

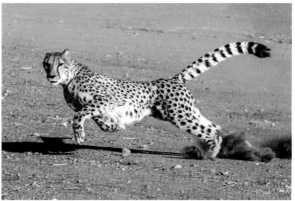

ABOVE
A running cheetah clearly shows flexion and extension movement patterns.

LEFT
Rotation forms a fundamental part of our gait, most clearly demonstrated by Olympic runners.

healthy children will express them at some point as part of the process of learning to sit, crawl and walk.

In addition to this, if we look around the world and see how different cultures go about their everyday tasks, we can get an impression of the sort of movements that people use regularly and repeatedly. And if we see that there is a commonality about the way people around the world move, we can draw tentative conclusions about how we are adapted for certain things. These days, the internet makes our job easier; a cursory look online for images of movement such as bending, sitting, etc. reveals a remarkable level of coherence.

What all of these studies tell us is that the history of our species has shaped us in a particular way, a way that supports certain movements well. It means we have *resilience* to these kinds of movements, because we are anatomically well adapted for them. If we are well adapted for them, they are likely to be safe. Conversely, if the movements we teach in yoga have no relationship to the movements shown either by evolution or by childhood development, we need to ask whether we are resilient to those movements if we repeat them regularly. Are they actually useful? I would argue, for example, that the Iyengar-style Triangle pose (Trikonasana) is potentially harmful (and thus arguably pointless), as are asanas such as Paravritta Janu Sirsasana and Warrior Two.

MOVING YOGA FORWARD

Those who practise yoga on a regular basis know that something positive happens; this is the undeniable experience of many. But what actually happens when we practise? The benefits fall into three main categories: benefits to the neuromuscular system, expressed through a greater sense of ease during movement at the joints and muscles of the body; an improvement in the responsiveness of the respiratory system, enabling it to meet the needs of changes in effort, emotions and posture; and finally a greater sense of wellbeing that has something to do with the way we engage with the nervous system – both in the way we respond to our internal, physical promptings (hunger, thirst, tiredness etc.), and to our external, social promptings (in connection with relationships, community and the environment).

These three categories overlap considerably: improvements in movement tend to improve breathing, improvements in breathing can help movement, and both will have an effect on our sense of wellbeing.

When we teach or practise yoga, we can reflect on the movements human beings make and ask ourselves if what we are doing falls into these categories. Yoga has traditionally had families of asanas – forward bends, back bends, side bends, twists, seated postures and balances – that are useful. These all still have a place in the modern lexicon of human movement if they are approached intelligently and if we are clear about the larger

intention of our posture work. If we are teaching a back bend like face-up Dog pose, we are examining how well the whole body expresses the movement. We are trying to discover if the whole body understands how to extend or whether it is only the neck and lower back that participate. We will notice how the uptake of certain muscles in back-bending necessarily changes our breathing pattern, rather than trying to impose a breathing pattern on the movement (as discussed more in chapter three). We will see similar things in flexion movements like squatting, where the shape of the body and its orientation to gravity will have a predictable effect on the breath. What we want to find out is whether the body adapts the breathing to the pose effectively or not. What we do not want to do is to try and control the breath in some supposedly idealised way while we practise.

'In flexion movements like squatting, the shape of the body and its orientation to gravity will have a predictable effect on the breath.'

Having taken a critical look at the way posture work has been approached in many systems of yoga, and suggested other ways of viewing movement and the body, in the next chapter I want to flesh out a more integrated way of approaching the subject. I will take a step back and look at the broader role of muscles, bones and fascia, and argue in chapter three that breathing and movement are inseparable aspects of our nature and need to be viewed together as integrated systems, not as individually discrete ones.

RIGHT
Squatting comes naturally to most children – a movement pattern that continues into adulthood in some cultures.

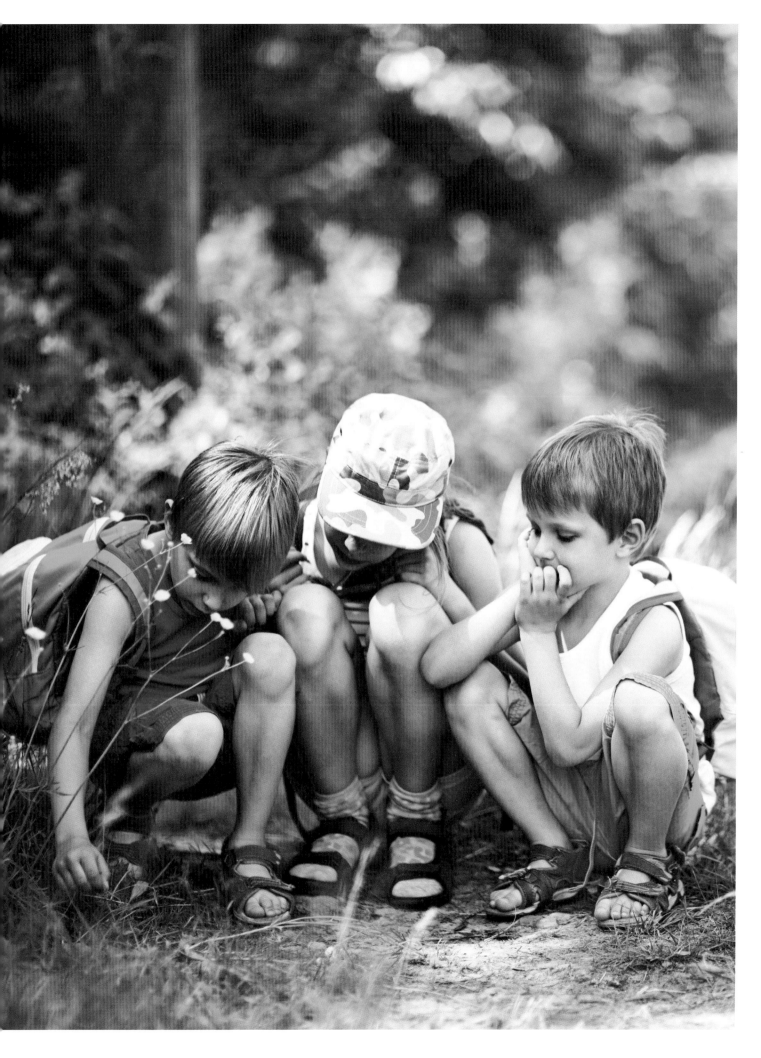

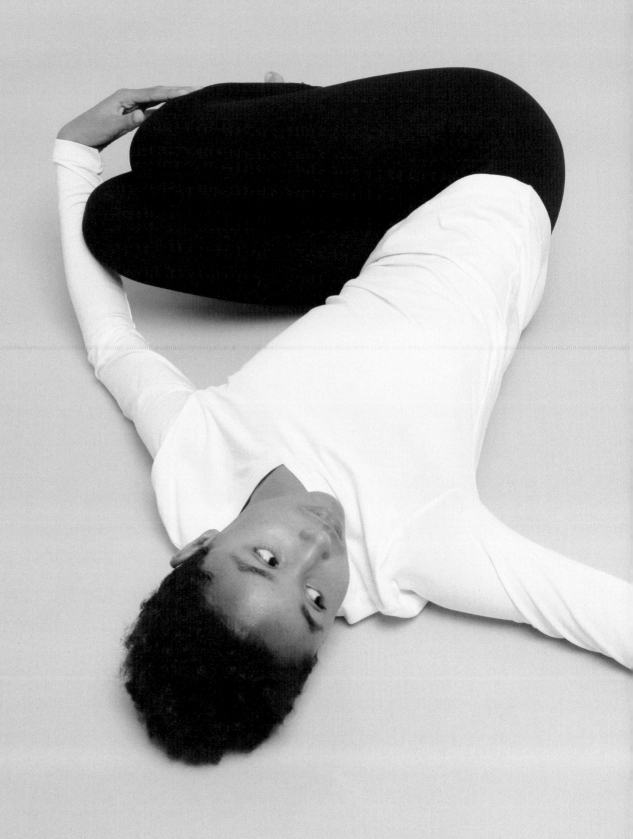

—— TWO ——

THE NEURAL BODY
Mapping movement patterns

We are neurological creatures. Information flows into us through our senses, is processed in our brains and then responded to through our muscles, cells and glands. How we *process* the information will vary from person to person and culture to culture. Consequently, our *responses* to information will also vary from person to person and culture to culture. For example, a child growing up in a big rumbustious family used to noise and people may enjoy the hustle and bustle of city life – or at least not be daunted by it; however, quietness and solitude may provide a challenge. Conversely, an only child brought up in the quiet of the countryside may feel overwhelmed by city life but comforted by quiet walks in nature. Our response will be noticed in our muscles, which will tend to tighten when our environment discomforts us, and relax when it nourishes us.

We see these muscular responses to the world written into our bodies as we age. To some extent, they define who we are – they create predictable responses to life's events. But there can be a downside, and that is that the responses we developed in early life may not serve us so well in our current situation. How we unpick the helpful habits from the unhelpful ones is a large part of our yoga practice, and this book deals with ways of approaching this elusive but important aspect of our being.

THE DEVELOPING MOTOR SYSTEM

In the beginning we are all much the same. When a baby is born, its voluntary motor control is almost nil; it is impossible for a baby to do anything it wants. Indeed, it may not even know what it wants, other than to survive. To help it to survive, the nervous system is partially 'hard-wired' at birth, with breathing and the heartbeat occurring automatically, but this is not enough to ensure survival. The baby also needs to eat, and so it arrives with a rooting instinct: an ability to nuzzle in search of the nipple and, once it finds it, to suck. In fact, the instinct to suck is so strong that anything placed near the baby's mouth will initiate a sucking response. The voluntary muscles of the mouth come pre-programmed; these are the survival reflexes – specific, predictable responses that are not under the control of the conscious mind, but which are elicited by a particular stimulus – without which a baby would soon die.

The muscular system also has more general reflexes, more survival programmes, albeit ones active in the longer term. These are reflexes that help coordinate the muscular system in response to gravity. Some are more local, like the grasping reflex of the hands and feet, while others are more global, using most of the muscles of the trunk. They develop the sequential strength in the muscles needed for locomotion. They include coordinated movements of flexion, extension, side-bending and rolling.

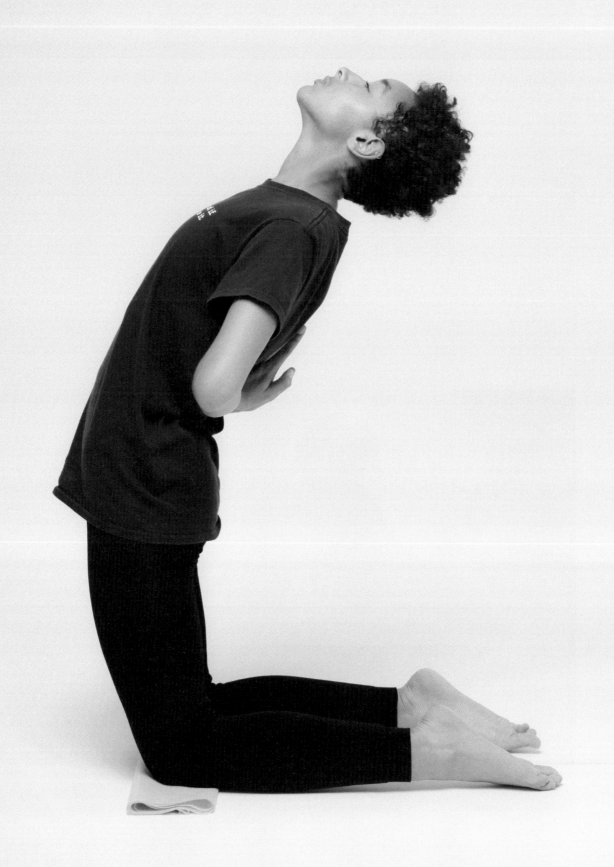

As the nervous system matures, these reflexes begin to become integrated into the infant's motivations and form the basis for volitional movement. He or she may want to follow the movements of a parent or, later, to pick up a toy. Ideally, reflexes enable the will to be acted upon, and it seems important that a child is given enough time to fully integrate them. Any encouragement to speed the process up by trying to get infants to sit, stand or walk before they find the necessary preceding steps may well come at some cost to their later motor skills.

The desire for movement integrates the reflex responses into functions such as crawling, creeping, sitting and eventually standing and walking. How successful this progression is will depend to a large extent on the emotional climate in which a child is growing. A safe, loving environment will provide the ideal background for integrated motor development. If the child is made anxious at this time, the tension this causes in the baby's muscles will interfere with the development of easy movement.

HABITUATED MOVEMENT AND 'BODY MAPPING'

As the child grows, it will habituate the things it does most often: running, walking, bending, sitting and a whole host of other movements that it does on a daily basis. How successful we are at habituating movement depends to some extent on need. We tend to perfect a task well enough to accomplish a desired outcome. Take handwriting, for example. Very few of us perfect our handwriting. We stop trying to improve it when it can be easily read and easily written, and this is true of almost any habit,

BELOW
Children have an instinctive desire for movement.

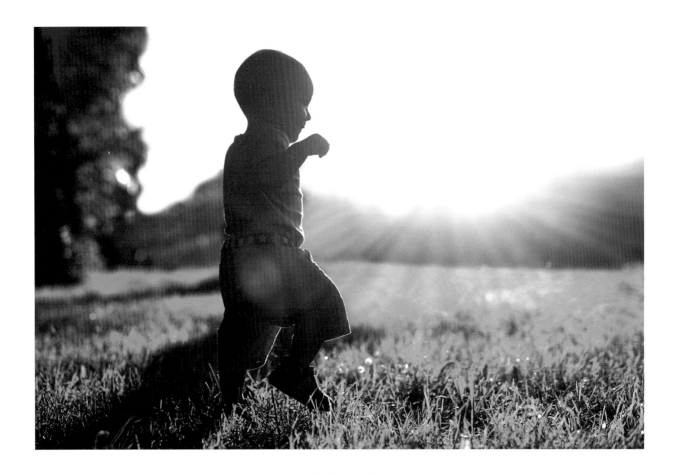

including running and walking. If we were still hunter-gatherers, we would spend much more of our lives perfecting these actions through necessity, but these days most of us can get by with relatively poor movement skills, and this is one of the reasons that we become more awkward and less confident in our movements as we age.

Habituation is a vitally important process that allows us to act speedily while at the same time keeping our conscious brain clear for more pressing activities. How we learn to habituate movement is a process called 'body mapping'. Anything we do regularly will become 'mapped' in the somatosensory part of the brain (a process that has been understood with the help of the advent of FMRI imaging of the brain over the last twenty years). It is useful to remember this when we practise yoga – that when we repeat movements regularly we begin to map them into our brains.

It makes sense, then, to map movements that are useful in life. These movements might include bending, turning, sitting, looking up etc. What is important when considering yoga from this perspective is that we are clear about what our intention is: what movement are we trying to practise and how well are we managing the movement? This approach contrasts with a way of practising that focuses on trying to stretch or strengthen a particular muscle or group of muscles, or even free a particular joint. As we shall see, the brain does not organise itself around discrete body parts, it only deals with *whole movement patterns*.

THE HISTORY BEHIND THE CONCEPT

Our understanding of body mapping has changed significantly in the last fifteen years, and it is useful to visit the history of this science briefly as it is germane to the discussion outlined above.

Historically, nearly all anatomy has been studied through dissection, and from this practice it was not unreasonable to ascribe certain movements to the muscles that anatomists found under the skin. Leonardo da Vinci, who did detailed dissection drawings, preceded Isaac Newton by more than a hundred years, but much of the anatomical research

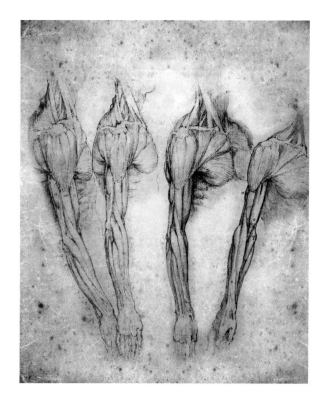

ABOVE
The mechanistic human machine: Leonardo da Vinci's detailed dissection drawings.

that went on after Leonardo was done against the backdrop of the mechanistic discoveries of Newton and those that followed him. The mechanistic human machine was a powerful idea.

These ideas were given further impetus in the latter part of the nineteenth century, when areas of the brain were found to control certain muscles. There was much debate about how parts of the cerebral cortex controlled movement, but the argument seemed to be settled when, in 1947, Wilder Penfield, after painstaking research, published his map of the motor and sensory cortex. Perhaps because he took the step to publish it in a pictorial way, it stayed in the imagination of those who study the nervous system in a way words never could. Penfield encountered a frustration, though: however carefully he stimulated the discrete areas of the motor cortex (of partially anaesthetised patients), he frequently found himself getting agitated over the responses – a muscle he did not expect to move

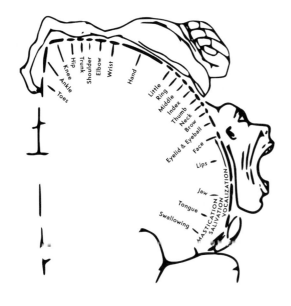

ABOVE
Wilder Penfield's homunculus diagram of
the sensory and motor regions of the brain.

would move. He put this down to his equipment, which he felt was not sufficiently delicate, resulting in an overlapping of stimulation.

However, in 1971, H. Asanuma, a scientist with much more sophisticated equipment, tried to map the motor cortex even more accurately. Using micro-stimulation techniques with ultra-fine wire electrodes, he tried to stimulate one neuron at a time, hoping to find an absolute one-to-one relationship between motor cortex areas and individual muscles. He was looking for a twitch response in the muscle stimulated. Even then – and somewhat frustratingly for an experimenter out to prove a point – a small amount of overlap still occurred. What Asanuma and Penfield before him had set out to prove was that if you stimulated a neuron in the motor cortex, the impulse would travel down the nerve and excite the muscle at the other end. The analogy of throwing a light switch and the bulb lighting up is obvious, and appealing.

All this research was thrown into question in the late 1990s. As often happens, an accidental laboratory observation revealed a very different possibility in the way the motor cortex is laid out. A researcher had been attempting to research the frontal eye field with an electrode stimulation that lasted for half a second rather than the much briefer five milliseconds used to study the motor cortex. Inadvertently he had missed the frontal eye field and got the electrode into the primary motor cortex. When the half-second stimulation was applied, the monkey extended its arm forwards and shaped its fingers as if to reach for something. *A whole movement pattern unfolded.*

These observations led to a new line of research where stimulation was extended somewhat to see what happened. The results were astonishing and led to an overturning of the discrete muscle theory. What Michael Graziano, Tirin Moore and Charlotte Taylor discovered – documented in Graziano's book, *The Intelligent Movement Machine: An Ethological Perspective on the Primate Motor System (2009)* – was that the motor cortex is mapped onto behavioural repertoires. The stimulation of one neuron does not lead to a downward pulse along the line of the nerve to the muscle; rather it spreads out to recruit other neurons, causing a whole group of muscles to be recruited into a recognisable movement pattern. What previous researchers had noted as a discrete muscle twitch was in fact the tip of a movement iceberg. It was the pursuit of an anticipated concept – direct neuron-to-muscle relationships – that had stopped them seeing the overlaps they were getting for what they really were: the start of a behavioural movement pattern.

We now know that the motor cortex 'maps' movement patterns that are frequently used. Nowhere is there a one-to-one relationship from motor neuron to muscle. As yoga teachers, this

RIGHT
We think and feel as a whole unit, and this is
reflected in our learned movement patterns.

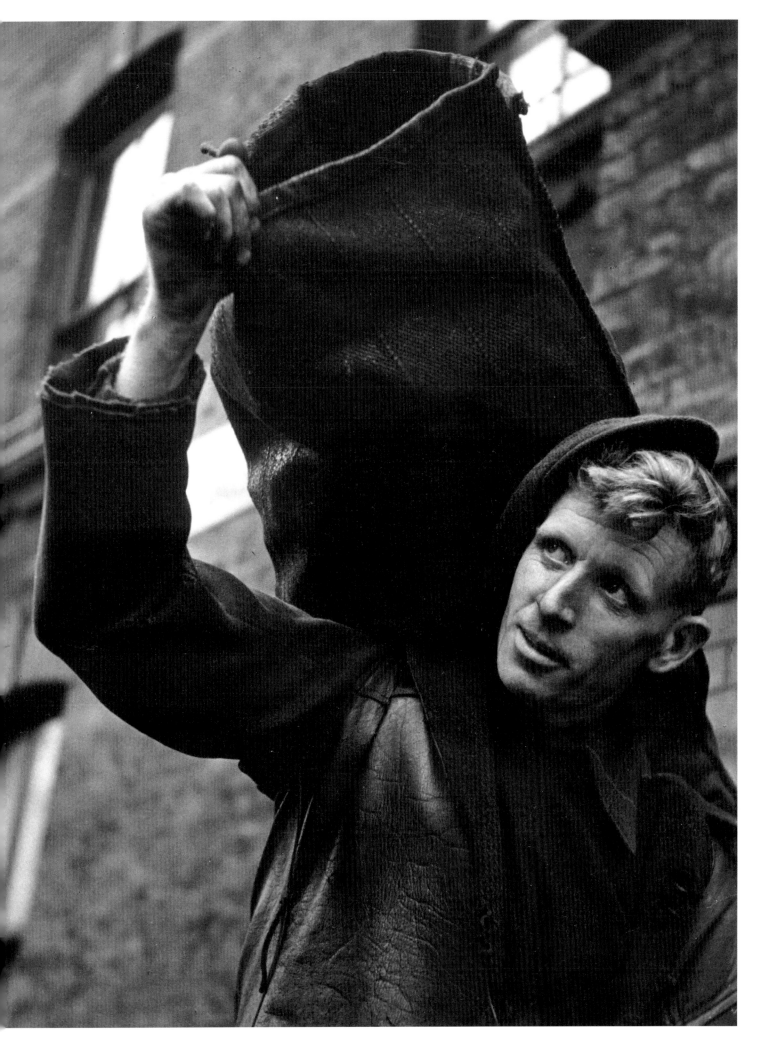

should make us think. Is there any point in trying to target specific muscles when the brain is not adapted for it? We should instead think in terms of functional movements, as described in chapter one and in the practical asana section of this book, or in terms of Graziano's 'behavioural repertoires'. The distinction between these two terms is very blurred; it could be argued that functional movements reflect evolution – so, movements of locomotion, feeding and reproduction – while behavioural repertoires might include more adaptive actions that are not directly related to survival. However, the terms are often interchangeable. What is important is that, whatever term is used, the whole body is asked to participate, not discrete muscles.

BELOW
A child learns to ride a bike through a process of feeling and habituation.

WHOLE BODY MOVEMENTS

Functional thinking is concerned with how we move as a whole when we carry out an intention. The intention may be straightforward – simply walking, sitting or picking something up off the floor – but these will be whole body movements, resulting from a flood of nervous impulses permeating the musculoskeletal system. The impulses initiate a sequence of muscular events that result in the desired action. The significant thing here is that we do not think about these movements as discrete parts that we have to coordinate. We think and feel as a whole unit.

This approach is natural, in the sense that all children learn to move like this, as do all animals. Even when we learn a new skill, like riding a bike, we do it as a whole person, and we do it by feeling. Movement is learned through our sensory nervous system. If we lose the sensory nerves, as can happen in some illnesses (graphically described by Oliver Sacks in his book *The Man Who Mistook his Wife*

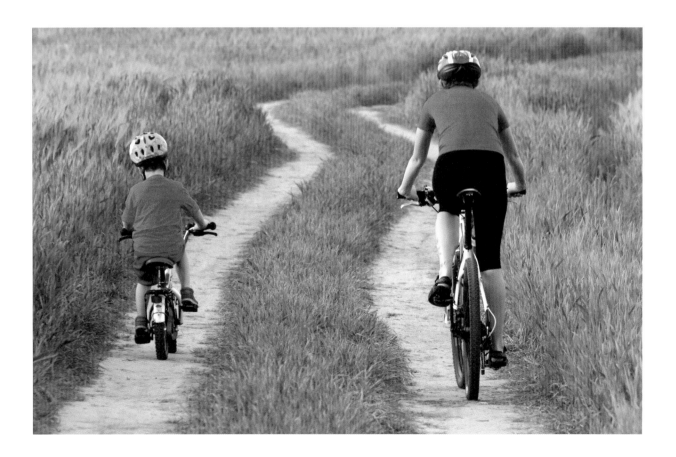

for a Hat), we no longer know how to move. This is because movement is dependent on sensory feedback to know where we are in space. Without this knowledge, a muscle can move you but it will not 'know' where it is moving you, so movements look flailing and uncoordinated (Oliver Sacks' 'disembodied lady'). This is not true of the motor nerves. If we lose a motor nerve, other pathways will open up to try to compensate; we will still know how to move, even though the action may be weaker because we have lost the use of a particular muscle.

The learning of a habit like driving or walking takes practice, and we continue practising until the action can be carried out successfully with little thought. This is different from habits of tension that creep into us because of our individualised responses to stress. We do not consciously practise these responses, but they become as normal to us as those we do practise. What we see in people are their learned movement patterns with their distinctive holding patterns overlaid on them.

COMPLIANCE AND DIFFERENTIATION

It is important to recognise the impact that acquired tension has on our volitional movements. If we are lucky enough to be unencumbered by tension in our muscles, our movements will tend to be free and efficient; our whole body will partake usefully in any action carried out. When a movement is carried out in such a way it is considered to be *compliant* – the body complies with the person's wishes in the easiest possible way. If, on the other hand, we have gathered tension in our muscles because our life has been less easy, we might find that one part of our body does not move as freely as another. For instance, we might lift our arm and the whole shoulder girdle lifts at the same time, and in a case like this we can say that there is a lack of *differentiation* between the arm (the humerus) and the shoulder girdle and trunk.

To develop fully compliant movements, our body needs to be well differentiated, and much of our yoga practice should be around developing differentiation in our joints (i.e. where one bone meets another) to enable us to make fully compliant

'We can improve our everyday movements by paying attention to the way we do them and consequently mapping them more accurately into our sensory motor cortex.'

————

movements in life in general. As practitioners of yoga, we can learn to do two main things in terms of movement. Firstly, we can improve our everyday movements by paying attention to the way we do them and consequently mapping them more accurately into our sensory motor cortex. Secondly, we can learn to become aware of the unintended tensions our individual lives have woven into us and, through careful practice, free ourselves of this encumbrance from our past.

YOGA AND THE NERVOUS SYSTEM

As I explained in chapter one, yoga, as I approach it, is firstly concerned with trying to restore what we could loosely call 'normal human movement'. Secondly, we are trying to help people notice the unacknowledged tension they bring to their movements. Thirdly, we are trying to improve the compliance (through differentiation) of the body by mapping all areas as richly as possible. And, finally, we are trying to help people notice when they move from a situation of comfort into one of discomfort, be it on a physical, psychological or even a philosophical level.

All these things which we are trying to observe in ourselves are aspects of our nervous system, our awareness of who we are and how we respond to the world around us. To change these things, we need to engage with exactly this part of our nature. Our anatomy is, of course, important (see pages 48–51) – we want our bodies to be functioning well so we can act unhindered by them. But it is misleading to think that we bring about change by trying to change our anatomy. Instead, we bring about change by changing that which acts on our anatomy – that elusive thing we call our 'self'.

THE NERVOUS SYSTEM AND HUMAN ANATOMY

Movement, as I've argued in this chapter, is a neurological event and an act of practice more than anything else. But, as our nervous system acts on our anatomy, having a relevant understanding of our anatomy can be extremely useful.

There are three major components to our anatomy that are of particular interest to us as yoga teachers (and students): muscles, fascia/connective tissue and bones. In a very straightforward way we can say that muscles generate forces to move us, fascia resists tensile forces and shapes us, and bones transmit forces to take the burden off muscles.

MUSCLES

The primary role of muscle in the body is to generate forces. Those forces are used for various tasks, movement being an obvious one, but also, of course, the tasks of breathing, digestion and circulation from the heart. Here I will focus on skeletal muscle, which we are most familiar with in our yoga practice.

Muscles are highly responsive tissues with a direct connection to the nervous system. They enable us to act out our wishes through their connection to the cortex, and are the only way we can respond voluntarily to the world.

The separation of muscles into named compartments is a geographical convenience but functionally misleading. When we decide to do something there is never a moment when we choose which discrete muscles we should use; instead, we orchestrate our nervous system as a whole. When we practise a movement regularly, we know that the nervous system maps the movement and if we pay close attention to the way we do the movement it will tend to become easier. This involves a change in the nervous system. The neurons in the sensorimotor cortex involved in the movement strengthen the pathways for useful muscular activity and prune away the connections that cause unhelpful muscular activity. This is how

the movement map improves. However, if the movement requires a lot of effort to perform – say, cycling up a steep hill – other changes will take place. Initially there will be an increase in the capillary network to the muscles involved, to ensure an improved blood supply to the muscles that have to do the hard work. So, the first adaptations to exercise are in the nervous system and the blood capillary network. If this is not enough to meet the needs of the activity, the muscle itself may grow bigger. Generally a muscle will only increase in size if the work it is being asked to do gets steadily harder, which is why body builders have to keep increasing the size of their weights. If they kept the weight at the same size but increased the repetitions, the muscle would not grow much bigger – it would be the capillary network that would increase. It is wonderful how specifically the body responds to its needs.

The other change, which yoga practitioners are particularly familiar with, is the increase in range of movement. There is little doubt that if you practise yoga regularly, your range of movement can improve significantly. However, there is some confusion over how exactly this happens.

In the past, it was thought that when we regularly stretch, the muscle and connective tissue grow longer and that is how we gain flexibility. But in the last fifteen years, much doubt has been cast on this theory, and more recently it has been suggested that changes in our range of movement are largely neurologically mediated. It seems that how much we are able to stretch a muscle is due to the signals we get from the sensory nerve endings in and around the muscle. These send messages to the brain, creating a default setting based on how much we generally stretch that muscle. When we go beyond that level of stretch, our nervous system notices and flags it up as unusual and we notice it as an increasing feel of stretch. However, if we start to stretch regularly, we 'reset' the default setting and our nervous system allows us to move a bit further than we could previously before giving us the signal that we are stretching.

There is an interesting footnote to the changes

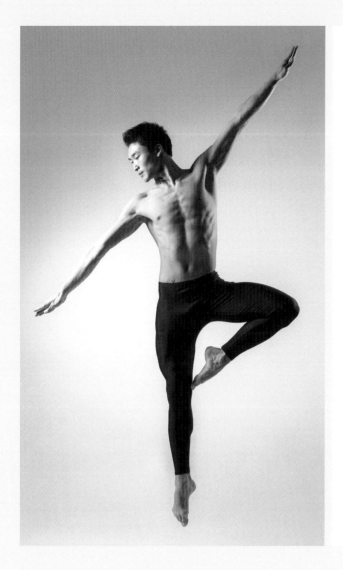

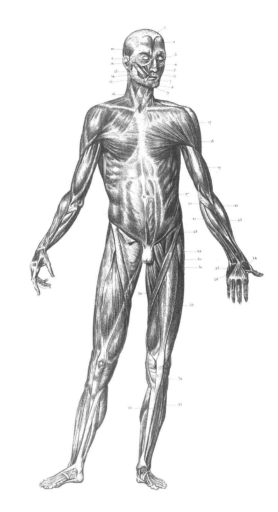

ABOVE
Whole body movement versus the misleading
separation of muscles into named compartments.

that take place in us when we start to exercise, and
that is that there is a great variation in our responses
to exercise. Some people gain muscle easily, others
do not; some develop aerobic capacity quickly, some
remain stubbornly resistant to training. And though it
has not been studied so extensively, I suspect some
people increase their range of movement more easily
than others. The non-responders to exercise are a
significant minority, in some studies as high as 18 per
cent. This is one of the reasons I increasingly feel it
is a mistake to think of yoga as an exercise system.
If you do think of it as exercise you will inevitably
exclude this group of people, who will simply feel
dispirited by their lack of improvement.

FASCIA/CONNECTIVE TISSUE
A great deal has been written about this fascinating
tissue over the past twenty years, the most
striking aspect being its all-encompassing nature.
Connective tissue surrounds almost every aspect
of our body. The only parts of us that escape its
grip are our teeth, nails and hair. It surrounds our
muscles, where it is called the *epimysium*, and joins
them to bones, where it becomes *tendons*. Where it
envelopes bone it is called the *periostium*; where it
joins bone to bone it is termed *ligament*.

If you could dissolve away every part of the body
but the fascia, you would be left with an intricate and
elaborate human-shaped lattice, with every internal
recognisable structure having its own particular
mesh. If we did the reverse and removed the entire
fascia matrix from a human being, we would become
a rather unappealing gooey, shapeless blob on the

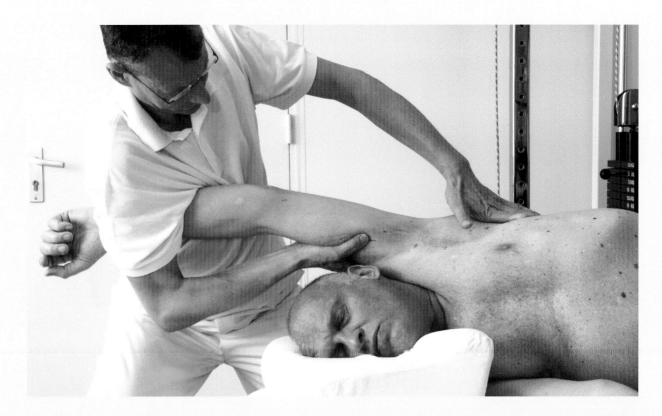

ABOVE
Rolfing is a deep manual therapy that works
on the fascia to try to balance the body.

floor, with our bones sticking out.

Every time we bend or stretch it is the fascial
system that feels it and gives us that sensation of
stretch that we are familiar with. This is because
this tissue is richly populated with sensory nerve
endings. Over the last two decades there has been
a lively debate around how much fascia can be
changed by manual therapy or through exercise,
and proponents of deep manual therapies like
Rolfing, or of forms of yoga that feature strong,
sustained stretching, believe that these things can
have a permanent impact on the length of fascia.
But recent research – for example, studies based on
the work of Robert Schleip at the Fascia Research
Project in Germany – throws quite a bit of doubt on
this, and many informed people have moved away
from this idea.

One thing that is unarguable about fascia is that
it is rich in sensory nerve endings, with interesting
and exotic names, such as the 'golgi' receptors
that surround joints, the 'pacini' receptors found
in tendons, spinal ligaments and some muscle

tissue, and the 'ruffini' receptors found in the
dura mater and the ligaments of peripheral joints.
More recently a whole new network of nerves has
been discovered, with nerves that are smaller but
much more abundant. These have been named
'interstitial receptors', though their role is not yet
fully understood. What is absolutely clear, though,
is that the point of sensory nerve fibres is to impart
information to the rest of the body and the brain.
Whether we are clear about the exact role they play
does not matter as much as the recognition that
there is a great deal of information to be listened to.
So, the better we hear what our body has to say, the
better we can respond to its promptings.

BONES
Bone itself is not a neurological tissue. However,
when we use our bones effectively, we notice the
reduction of effort via the nervous system.

The role of bones is often overlooked in
movement. We see bones simply as useful
structures to which we can attach muscles, giving
those muscles more leverage to exert their power.
And they do do this. But another aspect of the role
of bones is the capacity for them to transmit forces
to the ground – namely, the force of gravity. In

yoga we sometimes call this 'grounding' (see p.100). It is a very important concept because when we find good support through our bones, our muscles are able to relax a little more. To put it another way, if a muscle cannot find support, it has to work to maintain its position.

A good example of this is when we move from being on all fours into Plank pose. When we are on all fours, the thigh bones support the pelvis in space, but when we remove them by straightening the legs, the muscles in the front of the body have to work really hard to maintain the position of the pelvis. When the knees come back under the pelvis, the muscles of the trunk can relax again.

Something similar goes on in standing. If we stand in Tadasana (Mountain pose), for example, we can imagine our thigh bones resting on our shin bones through the knee – the biggest joint in the body. Weight is then transmitted to the floor through the ankle and heel bones. There is very little muscular effort required. We certainly do not need to pull up our kneecaps to stand well. This is a waste of effort and shows a lack of understanding of the role of bones in support.

When our structure supports us well, we feel easier in the body. Our nervous system alerts us to the way we use ourselves and our structure has evolved to be made good use of.

THE ROLE OF THE NERVOUS SYSTEM

These three aspects of our musculoskeletal system – muscles, connective tissue and bones – support each other to make movement as economical as possible. They form a productive alliance against fatigue if we listen to their promptings and respond accordingly. If any one structure gets over-stressed, it will signal to us to move and allow another system to take over. It is the nervous system that orchestrates how we use our structure. The point, then, is to listen to its signals.

You can notice this if you walk home with a bag of shopping in your hand. You may start with your elbow straight and your arm down by your side; here the ligaments and tendons in your shoulder and elbow support the weight of the shopping, and

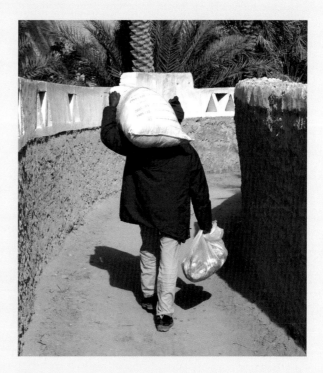

ABOVE
Carrying heavy bags involves a delicate interplay of muscles, connective tissue and bones, orchestrated by the nervous system.

the muscles do very little. After a while the stretch on those tissues will send you a signal that they are getting uncomfortable and you may be prompted to bend the elbow a little and lift the shoulder, thereby taking the strain off the connective tissue and handing it over to the muscles. This back-and-forth may go on for a few cycles, but at some point both may feel exhausted, so you may swing the bag over your shoulder to rest the weight on your collarbone, alleviating both muscle and connective tissue – until your fingers start to cramp and you decide to shift again.

The mistake that can sometimes be made in yoga is to give too much emphasis to any one system – usually muscles or fascia – in the mistaken belief that one system is somehow more important than another. Human beings are a complex interweaving of systems. No one system lords it over the others or should be given privileged status. If we want to exist in the world without unnecessary conflict, either within ourselves or in the wider world, then we need to develop the skill of noticing how we are feeling, and then deciding how to act on those feelings in the most intelligent way.

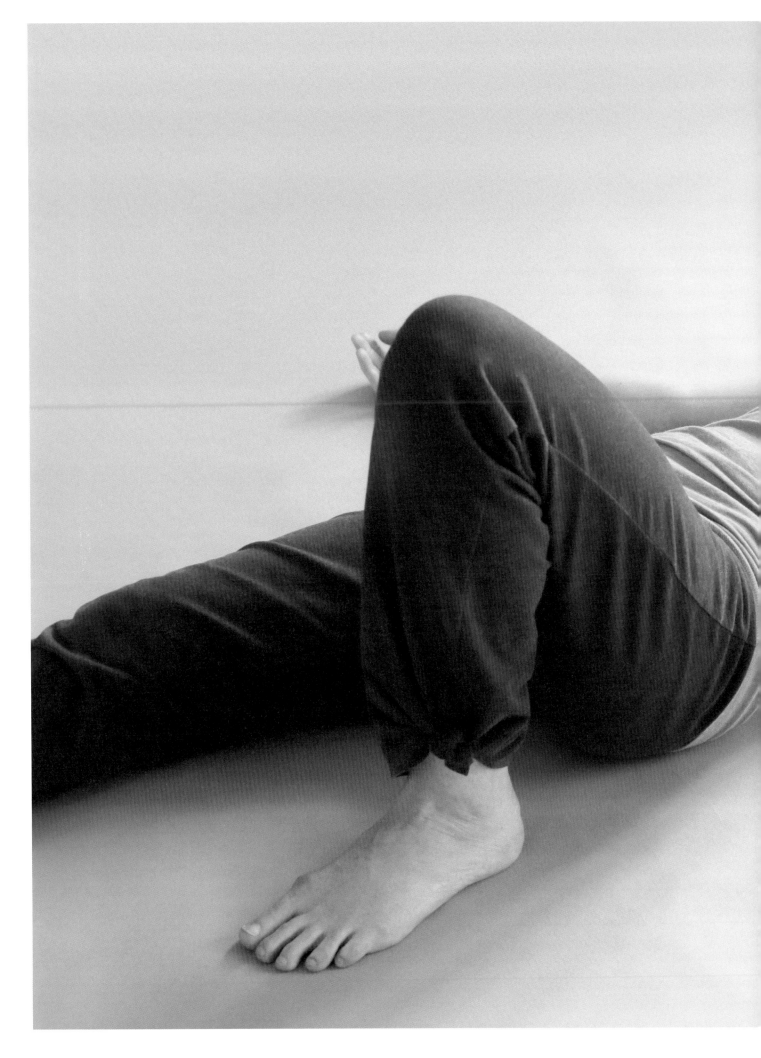

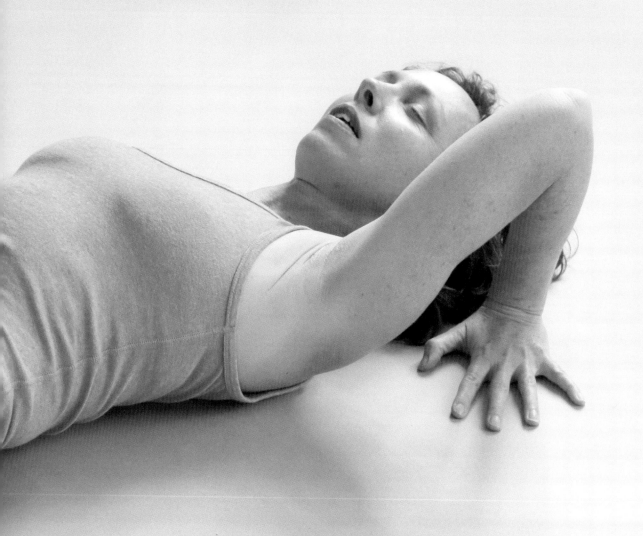

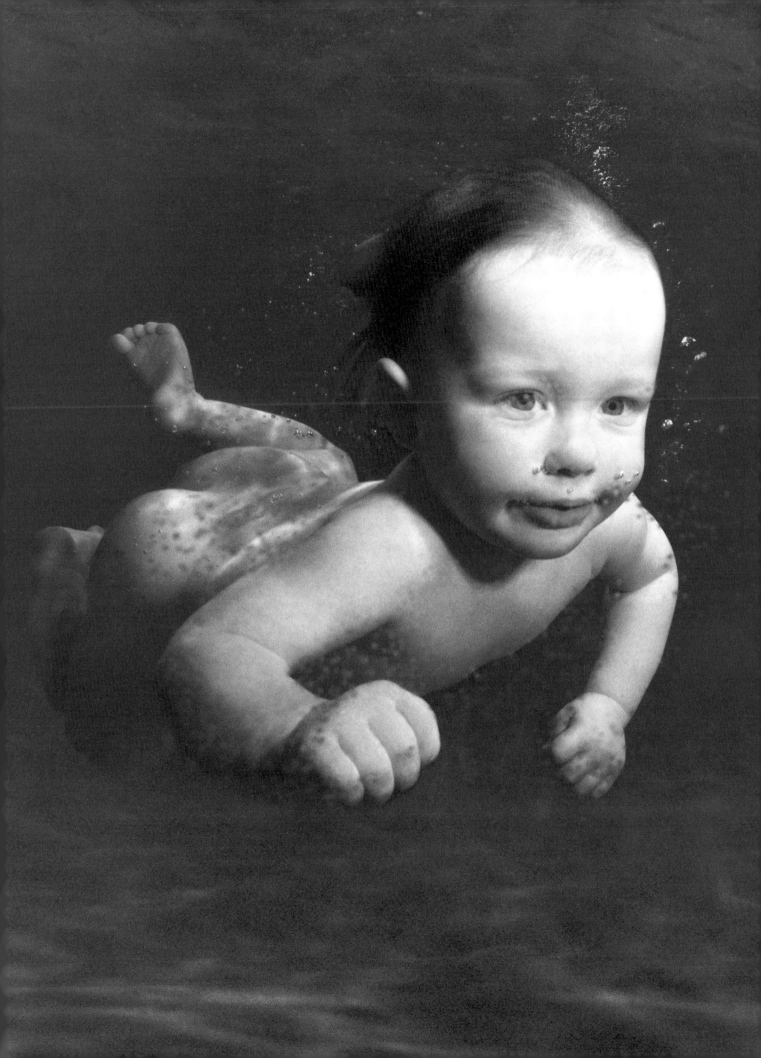

THREE

MAPPING BREATHING

Optimal respiration

Once we start to consider movement as something that is mapped rather than something that is governed by structure, it is relatively easy to see how we can reframe the physical side of yoga to incorporate a perspective that looks at whole body movement patterns rather than discrete parts of the body. However, it may not be so obvious that our breathing can be approached in the same way.

Breathing is often given special significance in yoga, because of its historical connection to *prana*; in fact, pranayama and breathing have almost become synonymous in some yoga circles. I think it is worthwhile distinguishing between the two. Pranayama deals with the esoteric concept of *prana*, or vital life force, and the practice of it involves ways of manipulating prana – with the end goal of enlightenment. This is a belief system that sits comfortably in the tantric tradition. It is not a belief I share. What I am interested in is *respiration*, and ways of making sure it is optimal under varying situations. Helping people notice the way the body self-regulates breathing, rather than imposing a preconceived idea of how and when we should breathe, seems more relevant to me. If breathing has gone awry for some reason, it is more helpful to try to understand what is interfering with the breath rather than adding another layer of conditioning to it. There are some techniques from pranayama

that are very helpful in freeing up the respiratory system, such as *Uddiyana bandha*, *Mula bandha* and *Kapalabhati*, which I use frequently. But I would like to reiterate that my use of these techniques is not with the intention of manipulating *prana* but rather to free up and 'map' unfamiliar ways of breathing.

RESPONSIVE BREATHING

The sensory cells (chemoreceptors) in the brain, and the carotid arteries in the neck, control the regulation of breathing by sending out messages to the muscles of respiration, asking them to allow breathing to happen in such a way that the body's equilibrium is maintained (homeostasis). In sleep and in rest the diaphragm is the major muscle involved; but when we are more active we will reach for additional muscles – muscles that we have learned to use, that we have 'mapped', throughout our life.

There are many things that can influence the way we breathe and therefore the muscles that get involved, and some are more obvious than others. The most obvious is exertion. The harder we work with our muscles, the more oxygen they require and the deeper we have to breathe. It is the carrying of oxygen through our bloodstream to our muscles that dictates the rate of breathing. If we have a powerful heart, one that has got larger

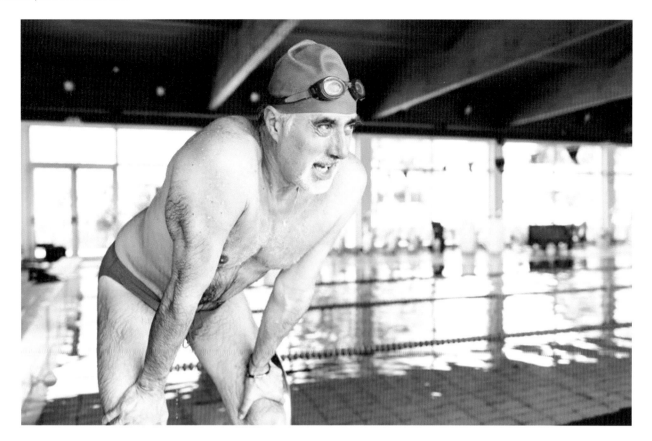

through regular aerobic exercise, we will need to breathe less frequently. If, on the other hand, our heart is compromised in some way – such as by a heart attack or a weakness in the valves – then small exertions, such as walking up the stairs, may result in laboured breathing. Similarly, if the iron (the haemoglobin, the carrier of oxygen in the blood) is reduced, as occurs in anaemia, we will breathe harder to try to compensate. These are examples of the way breathing automatically tries to compensate for a change in demand or a dysfunction elsewhere. An individual suffering from chronic problems, such as the ones described above, will tend to recruit accessory muscles of respiration much earlier than a healthy individual will. And these muscles will be recruited in the way a person has learned to use them over time. In these cases, it becomes even more important to try to identify anything unhelpful in these movements.

Our emotions also influence our breathing. The sighing, sobbing breath of grief is quite different from the short, fast breathing of excitement or anxiety. Grief demands of us that we lose tension. We might shake and sob with large releases of the diaphragm. The vulnerability of grief is marked by

our softening the venting of tension from almost every muscle. Anxiety and excitement, on the other hand, require us to pump blood into our muscles in preparation for action, so our breathing may speed up and the rib cage may become more involved as our abdomen tightens with anticipation. It is important for our emotional health that our body (and mind) are adaptable enough to express a full range of emotional states, and this is only possible if the emotional and physical 'maps' are there. The 'stiff upper lip' of the Victorian Englishman may have helped him survive the battlefield, but it left him far less well equipped to deal with the emotional outflow of such events. It is not helpful to tell our young boys that it is a sign of weakness to cry. It simply shuts down the possibility of venting feelings that arise and very likely leads to them being expressed in some other, often mysterious, way.

Less obvious and well documented than changes in breathing caused by physical exertion and emotional stress are those changes that occur with variations in posture and movement. It is noteworthy that many schools of yoga do not seem to acknowledge this, instead preferring to tell students when to breathe in or out in relationship to movement. This approach is unhelpful; far preferable is to help students understand how breathing changes with movement.

The fact that movement and breathing changes are intertwined is not news for our species. This has been the case ever since we first hauled ourselves out of the sea some 440 million years ago. We saw in chapter one how early lizards took with them the side-bending action of fish to move across the land, using the same muscles needed for breathing (the intercostals). Dogs also shift the function of their muscles according to need: standing still, the intercostals are used for breathing, but once a dog is running these muscles are recruited for locomotion and the diaphragm takes on the major role of respiration (the lizard would be jealous if it knew how much more effective this arrangement is). In fact, in a well-organised human body, each muscle is enrolled in the most pressing task at hand. Even the diaphragm may momentarily cease its respiratory excursions and help brace the thorax if a person is lifting something heavy.

Breathing requires a softness and freedom around the rib cage and belly. Any activity that demands that these muscles work for another task will to some extent compromise the breath. Try putting your body into Plank pose and then afterwards lying in semi-supine (on your back with your knees bent). It is clearly a little harder to breathe in the first posture. This is because in Plank our abdominal muscles are required to hold the trunk in place, so they consequently stiffen, making abdominal breathing less easy, and the ribs then tend to become more employed and breathing is thus more constrictive. In semi-supine, no muscles are required for action because the floor supports us. Thus breathing is unimpeded and the simplest breathing takes place – light abdominal breathing. Similarly, breathing changes will take place in a position like squatting, which tends to release the abdomen and

the pelvic floor, moving the breath more into the lower belly and making it more expulsive. That is why this position is traditionally used for giving birth or defecation.

It is clear that what we need is a respiratory system that can adapt to whatever situation it has to deal with, and that there is no such thing as a correct

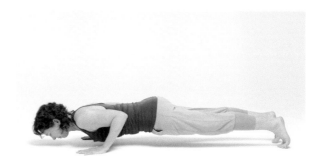

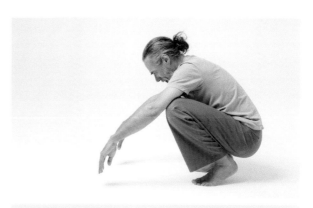

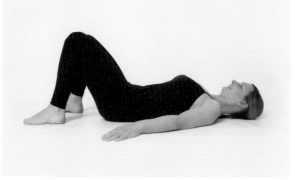

way to breathe or a 'yogic breath' that suits all occasions. We simply need to breathe in a way that is appropriate for the conditions we find ourselves in, and this should be an autonomic process, not a cognitive one. However, we often find – if we seek to notice – that we unintentionally compromise our breathing, and therefore our ability to respond optimally to life's demands.

When we practise yoga, our focus is not on imposing something on the breath; it is on refining our movements in such a way that the breath becomes free of the burden of the constraint of tense muscles. I have argued in earlier chapters that unconscious tension compromises compliant (efficient, whole-body) movement. It also compromises compliant breathing. The way out of the bind is to pay attention to our levels of support through our bones and the floor to reduce muscular tension, and learn to notice moment by moment when we are doing more than necessary. We particularly need to put aside any ideas around artificially pulling in the stomach, according to erroneous ideas about the 'core' or *bandhas*. Both concepts have been seriously questioned during the last decade. Studies examining claims made by proponents of core stability, in particular, have shown them to be largely false, with perhaps the most comprehensive criticism coming from Professor Eyal Lederman. Lederman's paper 'The Myth of Core Stability' (CPDO Online Journal, June 2007, pp1-17, www.cpdo.net) calls out the separation of 'core' and 'global' muscles as a 'reductionist fantasy', and states that core stability exercises are no more effective at preventing back pain than any other types of exercise.

'RE-MAPPING' OUR BREATHING

Perhaps our difficulty with understanding the ramifications of particular movements and related breathing patterns is because of the complex relationship that exists between the rib cage/thorax and the abdominal/pelvic chambers, which I will refer to respectively as the upper and lower chambers. Although the lungs only occupy the upper chamber, how well they can expand and contract does depend to a large extent on what is going on in the lower chamber. As mentioned above, an understanding of the interplay between the two chambers is significant for yoga practitioners because of ubiquitous erroneous ideas around maintaining bandhas or pulling in the 'core'. Breathing necessarily causes a continuous shape change in both chambers and this should not be artificially compromised. The lowering of the diaphragm on the inhalation tends to push downward on the abdominal and pelvic contents, which in turn pushes out the abdominal wall and pelvic floor. The box on pages 62–3 explains this more fully. This gentle rhythm is easy to see in the resting individual. At rest, abdominal ('diaphragmatic') breathing is the most energy-efficient way to breathe. All healthy people tend to breathe this way when resting, with a gentle rise and fall of the abdomen.

When we become active, however, our trunk muscles are required for other tasks, as described above, necessitating a change in breathing patterns. If we are well-embodied, with a rich and appropriate mapping of our movements, the interplay between breathing and movement will cause little conflict. Muscles will tighten to carry out an action and temporarily constrain the breath, but will relax again when the exertion passes and breathing gets restored to the most compliant possibility. We might see this if we try lifting a heavy object off the floor. The trunk muscles temporarily stiffen, and breathing becomes short or may even pause. Then, when the object is put down, the trunk muscles relax and breathing normalises.

In yoga this will happen every time we change postures. Coming from all fours to Plank will change our breathing, as the abdominals take over the work of the femurs to support the trunk in space. And in standing, if we look up into an extension movement, the abdominals reflexively tighten to support the spine, and breathing then

RIGHT
When we look down in flexion, our abdominal muscles relax as they're not required for action.

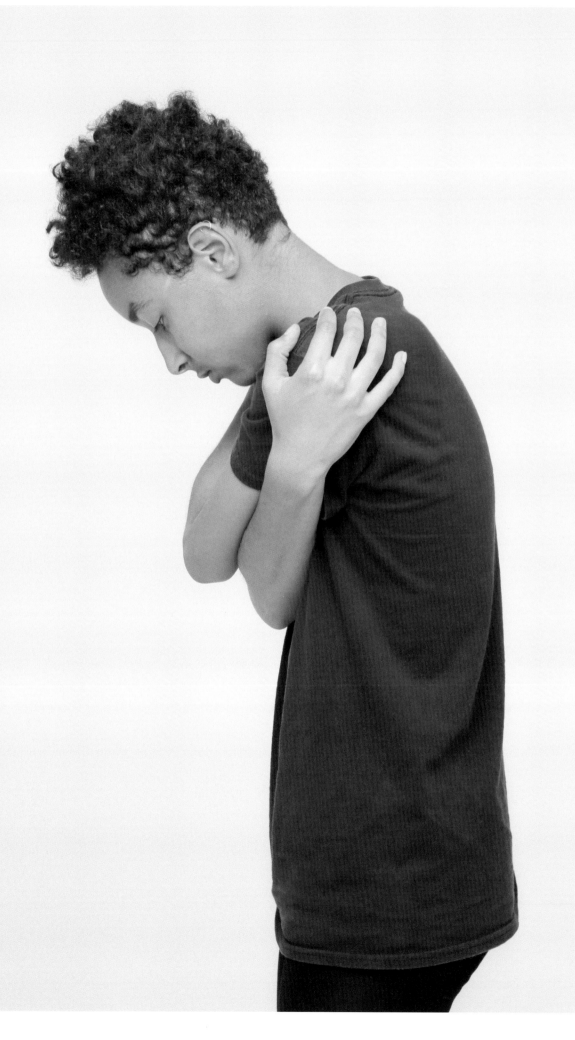

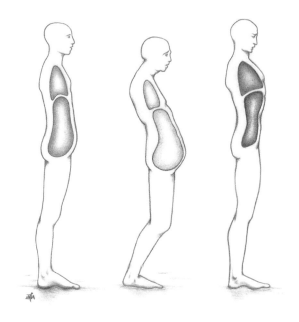

ABOVE
Habitually held tensions are behind common postural patterns, such as slumping or 'fronting up' to life.

necessarily moves up into the rib cage. If we then, following directly on from the extension movement, look down into flexion, the abdominals will relax because they are not required for this action. Gravity is adequate, and breathing will move down into the belly. Try doing these movements and see if you can observe the subtle changes. At this point we may find that cultural conditioning has taken over our response. Most people fear showing their tummy, and suck it in because of a cultural perception that it is unattractive. This adds another layer of interference to our natural breath.

So, what if we are poorly mapped? What if our grip on our muscles has become deeply habituated so that these unconscious but useful changes in shape and breathing do not take place so easily? Tensions that are habitually held in the diaphragm, the deep abdominal muscles or the muscles that elevate our ribs will interfere with the interplay between the upper and lower chambers that should exist in a healthy person, leading to a reduced ability to adapt breathing usefully, and to postural changes that embed such patterns further.

We see these changes in shape expressed in people we know and love every day. The person who pulls his shoulders back and draws up his breastbone whilst inflating the rib cage, like a soldier on the parade ground, is a fairly common sight in those who feel a need to 'front up' in life. Conversely, the sunken chest and swollen abdomen of the person who has lost all ability to meet life with resilience is shaped by respiration having moved down low into the abdomen. It is likely that this forms a negative spiral of events, where the slow changes in breathing and posture reinforce the emotional feelings that gave rise to them. The illustrations above, adapted from an image in Stanley Keleman's thought-provoking book *Emotional Anatomy,* published in 1985, give a few postural examples that may be familiar. If these rather fixed patterns dominate our daily lives, the ability to adapt function – to easily move between activities – becomes compromised.

Keleman argued that we go through various

somatic (bodily) stages in our response to increasing emotional stress, starting with resistance, often in the form of inflating ourselves through rigidity and fear, and ending with collapse and defeat if the stress continues to build. Each individual is caught somewhere on this spectrum if life is tough. If life gets safer we may unstiffen and choices will be freed up again. You can see these shape changes and the consequences imposed on the upper and lower chambers in those same drawings. It is clear, when you look at the drawings, that the most significant shape changes occur in the two chambers. It becomes apparent that there are two main players contributing to our posture, that are of course significantly related. If we stoop because our map of standing has become this way, and we are permanently in flexion, we are

> 'It is fruitless to try to change a breathing pattern until choices become available to a person in the way they stand and move.'

———

likely to be 'belly breathers' (the two go together as explained above). Similarly, if we have learned to hold ourselves upright through some cultural notion, or simply from bracing against the world, we will tend to be 'chest breathers'. It is fruitless to try to change a breathing pattern until choices become available to a person in the way they stand and move. To help bring forth these choices and thus free the breath, we have to be able to see the relationship between respiration and our postural holding maps, and to recognise that the maps of breathing can only change as our maps of moving and standing become richer and more nuanced.

'VISCEROPTOSIS' OF THE INTERNAL ORGANS
There is also another, slightly more contentious, aspect to the way the upper and lower chambers are 'held' through the way we map them. If the concept of body mapping is not clear here, then think of it as the way we habitually carry our rib cage and belly, linked to our pattern of breathing. We might be habitual belly breathers, habitual chest breathers, or anywhere in-between. It might not be a surprise to hear that people who inflate their rib cage and draw their abdomen in as a way of presenting themselves to the world tend to suffer with neck and shoulder pain, because of the amount of additional work these muscles are asked to do. However, it might be less obvious that someone whose abdomen has overly relaxed and whose diaphragm has tightened (patterns that are usually interlinked) often suffer from pelvic floor-related problems, including various forms of prolapse and herniation, because of the constant downward pressure. Not only that but when we either haul in our tummies or distend our abdomens as an unconscious response to the world, the organs that can move will shift position.

If this pattern continues over many years, it may have an adverse effect on the functioning of the organs involved. The relative position of the diaphragm and abdominal wall clearly affects the placement of the more mobile organs. One can speculate that the transverse colon, for example, will function better when appropriately positioned than when it is sagging. The kidneys, too, can migrate from the back of the body to the front of the pelvis, especially in thin people. It seems reasonable to assume that the more an organ is in the position it is supposed to be in, the better it will function. Downward pressure from the diaphragm will also push on the pelvic floor, and that may contribute to problems such as stress incontinence and prolapse.

This perspective has been on the fringes of healthcare over the last couple of centuries. In the late 1800s, the French physician Frantz Glénard took a great interest in visceroptosis – the sinking of internal organs below their natural position – as a cause of illness, as did the orthopaedic surgeon Joel Goldthwaite some fifty years later. In more recent times, visceral manipulation pioneered by the osteopath Jean-Pierre Barral has followed a similar line of thinking.

TECHNIQUES FOR RE-MAPPING BREATHING

Whether the muscular balance between the upper and lower chambers has been disturbed because of anxiety and stress or simply because constant sitting and little activity have weakened strategic muscles, the consequences can be far reaching. The normal homeostatic mechanisms outlined at the beginning of this chapter that regulate the breath can become disregulated, leading to breathing problems, muscular aches and pains, digestive issues and problems of the pelvic floor. Fortunately, yoga has a few tricks up its sleeve to help address these difficulties. It can be a wonderful way of restoring a helpful equilibrium when practised intelligently.

We have established that each chamber directly impacts on the other. We know that the primary function of the upper chamber is respiration, so it makes sense that the rib cage and diaphragm should be free and responsive enough for breathing to remain uncompromised. It is equally important that activity in the lower chamber does not interfere with the efficiency of the upper chamber, the thorax. This lower chamber needs to provide both postural and visceral support. It needs to be able to increase pressure enough for expulsive efforts, but must not interfere unnecessarily with the breath.

> 'Learning to release the exhalation fully helps release the diaphragm, preventing the build-up of tension.'

———

There are techniques in yoga specifically for redressing the balance between the upper and lower chambers. Learning to release the exhalation fully helps release the diaphragm, preventing the build up of tension. The bandhas ('locks' or 'bonds' in Sanskrit) exert a strong resistance to the downward pull of the diaphragm. *Mula bandha* – lifting up the muscles of the pelvic floor – maps the pelvic floor and the lower abdominal muscles, while *Uddiyana bandha* – lifting the diaphragm while pulling the

THE TWO CHAMBERS: A SYMBIOTIC RELATIONSHIP

To envisage these two chambers more clearly it is worth considering a few things. Firstly, the upper chamber has evolved to expand. It needs to expand in order to lower the pressure within itself. This expansion and consequent lowering of air pressure within the chamber causes air to flow down the pressure gradient from the outside to the inside, thereby inflating the lungs. The muscles that expand the rib cage can be seen in the drawing on the near right. The lower ribs move sideways and upwards in what is sometimes referred to as a bucket-handle action, while the upper ribs and the breastbone move forwards and upwards, in a pump-handle action. This difference is due to the way the lower and upper ribs attach to the spine. As we breathe in, the lower rib cage tends to widen, while the upper rib cage deepens.

However, that is not the only way the upper chamber can increase its volume. The floor of the chest wall is the diaphragm – a broad, dome-shaped muscle that spans the perimeter of the lower ribs, effectively separating the upper from the lower chamber. When we breathe in, the diaphragm contracts and lowers, thereby lowering the floor of the rib cage and adding volume by *vertically* deepening the upper chamber.

Whilst the upper chamber has evolved to expand and lower air pressure within, the lower chamber is the opposite. Its job is to maintain pressure and sometimes to increase it. In many ways the lower chamber is a relatively simple structure, as its main function is one of stricture. The deep abdominal muscle that forms the wall of the abdomen and pelvis, the *transverse abdominus*, is ideally suited for this task, as it forms an almost continuous structure with the diaphragm above and blends with the muscles of the inner wall of the pelvis below. With its horizontally aligned fibres, contraction

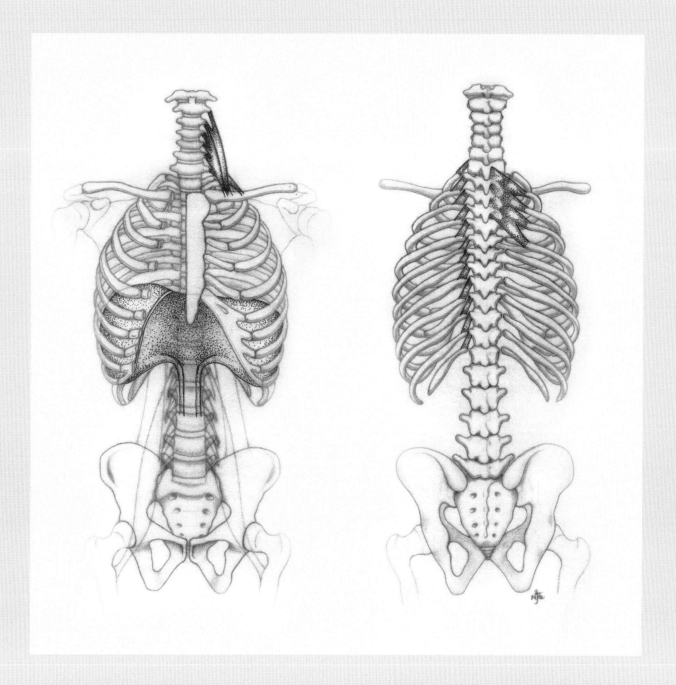

ABOVE
The muscles that expand the rib cage,
seen from the front and back of the torso.

of this muscle raises pressure in the abdomen and pelvis. This increase in intra-abdominal pressure is needed, firstly, as a means for expulsion – for excretion, vomiting, coughing and giving birth. But it also provides support, a fact that becomes quite obvious when we instinctively brace the abdomen when trying to lift a heavy object, and in so doing form a hydraulic column to protect the spine. In everyday life, support is also provided by the relative tensions of the abdominal muscular wall – mainly the transverse abdominus, the diaphragm and the pelvic floor. However, some clarification is needed about the relative roles played by the muscles of this wall, which can be divided into two main groups: those used for moving the skeleton, and those used to support the abdominal contents. The muscles used to move the skeleton are the external and internal obliques, and the *rectus abdominus*. The *transverse abdominus* supports the abdominal contents as well as increasing intra-abdominal pressure, as previously described.

upper abdominal muscles back towards the spine through the expansion of the rib cage – causes the diaphragm to be pulled strongly upwards, sucking both the abdomen, its contents (the internal organs) and the pelvic floor with it. These actions can play a part in preventing the positional displacement and compression of the abdominal and pelvic organs, and map the possible position of the diaphragm and all the concomitant changes it induces in the ribs and belly in more detail. If we add to this the practice of *Kapalabhati* (forced exhalation with a passive inhalation), we are then mapping the transverse abdominals and the pelvic floor, while the diaphragm is simultaneously encouraged to release. When we practise these things regularly, our respiratory map widens and becomes richer, allowing more potential for choice under life's varying circumstances.

Between them, these three yoga techniques are ideal for helping counteract the effects of gravity, the effects of diaphragmatic tension, and poor mapping of the respiratory system – all of which take their toll on the upright human body as we age. Of course,

these techniques focus on the muscles that are most directly related to respiration, and it would be folly to fail to recognise that the freeing up of the primary muscles of respiration needs to go hand in hand with the freeing up of the whole musculoskeletal system. Perhaps it is a false dichotomy to imply that they are separate at all because, as I have tried to show, respiration and movement have been closely linked for millennia. But I do think it can be useful to find methods that bring our attention to an area that can be difficult to notice. In much the same way that extra attention might be needed to wake up the feet (something I do in every class, with specific movements for the feet and particularly the toes), it can be helpful to find movements that draw our attention to the breath.

It is an interesting observation that when we truly start to lose tension and feel more free and less constrained in our movements, bandhas, particularly *Uddiyana* and *Mula bandha*, emerge in a natural way in certain postures. It could be said that if we notice Uddiyana 'arriving' when we practise Dog pose, for example, it implies that there is a useful freedom around the shoulders, rib cage and belly. This is in stark contrast to the engaging of a bandha during practice, which simply adds tension. Uddiyana requires a relaxed abdomen to allow it to draw in. It therefore tends to emerge when the belly is relaxed, which is when we do forward-bends from standing, or move towards Bridge from lying on our backs. It is the same for *Mula bandha*: the pelvic floor tends to draw up with the diaphragm as the diaphragm relaxes up. This may be made clearer by reviewing the way the two chambers relate, described on pages 62–3.

JALANDHARA BANDHA AND THE DEEP FLEXOR MUSCLES OF THE NECK

Jalandhara bandha can be looked at in a similar way to *Uddiyana bandha* and *Mula bandha*. To explain this, and how it can also help to free up our breathing, I need to digress to a subtle aspect of anatomy.

Some places in the body are difficult to visualise. They are also sometimes difficult to sense. One

BELOW
Uddiyana bandha can help to prevent downward compression of the organs.

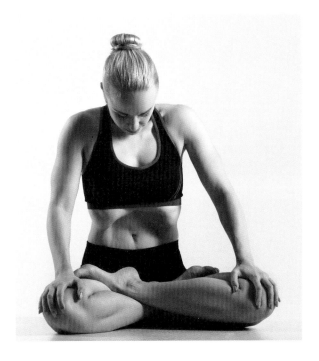

such place is where the spine meets the skull. This point is not under the chin, but more at the back of the palette – higher than you might imagine. It can be an interesting process to try to rest your attention here for a while. When we visualise this area, we can dwell on the small muscles that live high on the front of the spine: the *Longus colli* and the *Rectus capitis anterior*, small muscles that help balance the head on the spine where the atlas (the uppermost vertebra) meets the occiput (the base of the skull). These deep flexor muscles of the neck have the capacity to balance the large and very powerful muscles that extend the head on the spine.

If we just stand for a while and listen attentively to the 'voice' of the deep neck flexors, we might notice their gentle request for the front of the neck to draw in towards the back of the neck. The blustering neck extensors, because of their antagonistic role, then become slowly subdued. It is lovely to feel the sense of release of the skull from the neck, and to develop a 'nodding dog' feeling. This sense of depth within the neck is very useful in standing, and becomes even more important in the flexion movements.

The role these deep neck flexors perform takes the head and neck towards *Jalandhara bandha*, though not in the strong way described in some yoga books. It is something softer than that, a process that leaves the eyes relaxed and the nostrils quiet. This in itself takes the breath more towards *Ujjayi* – the way of breathing where the breath is felt at the back of the palette rather than the front of the nostrils, and the flow of air is slow and steady. Like *Uddiyana* and *Mula bandha*, *Jalandhara bandha* is the result of the subtle letting go of tensions in the body, and recognising this feeling is a confirmation that your practice is on the right track, that old habits are being left behind and new appropriate responses are being mapped.

BREATHING, THE SPINE AND NON-INTERFERENCE

There is one other aspect of breathing that is significant, and that is the subtle effect that breathing has on the relaxed spine. In the box on pages 62–3, I describe the action of the ribs to

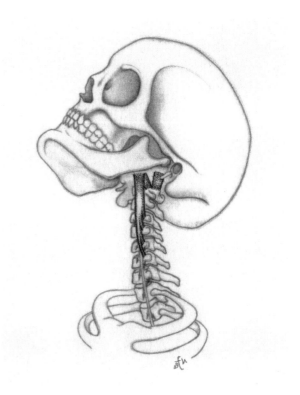

ABOVE
Paying attention to the deep flexor muscles of the neck can lead to a lovely sense of release.

increase the thoracic volume. There is, though, another aspect to the action of the ribs that is rarely mentioned in anatomy books, and that is the effect they have on the thoracic spine – how they effectively push the spine backwards into increased flexion on the inhalation. It is easy to confirm this by placing your hands on the thoracic spine of someone who is on all fours. You will quickly notice that the spine 'domes up' on the inhalation and flattens more on the exhalation. This gives the sense of the spine lengthening on the exhalation, which makes it logical for us to undertake extension movements on the out-breath rather than the in-breath.

When we pay attention to our breathing, it becomes clearer that the way we organise our bodies will have an effect on the way we breathe – and that breathing itself affects the body. The relationship is subtle and complex. Any clumsy attempts to prescribe ways of breathing or holding the abdomen will only interfere with this delicate interplay. Our best approach is to see if and where we interfere with the breath, and to do our very best to reduce that interference.

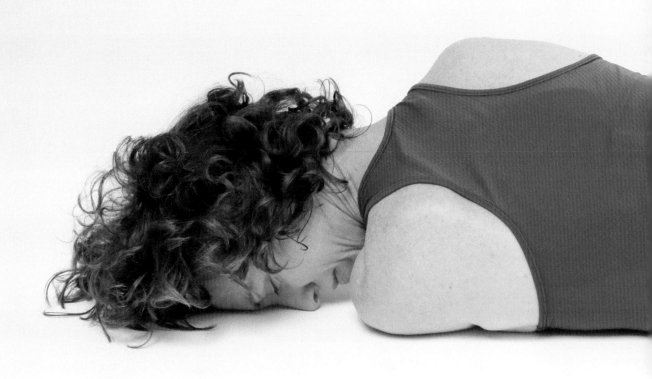

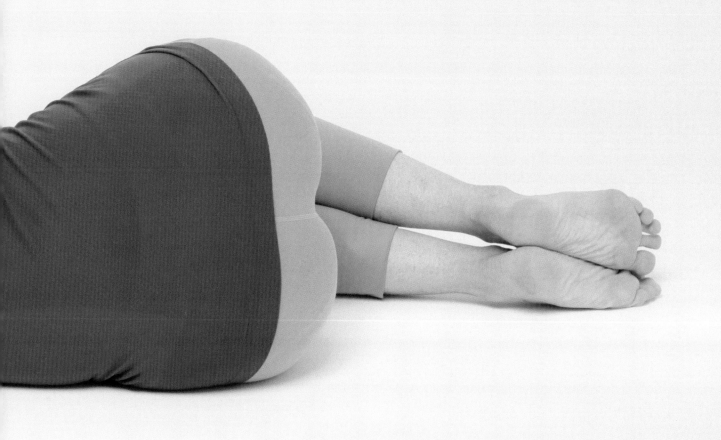

———— FOUR ————

WHEN THINGS GO WRONG

Dealing with chronic pain

I n the previous chapters of this book, I have emphasised the importance of paying attention to the sensations of the body – noticing how we feel and then responding to those feelings as appropriately as possible. However, there is one sensation that is normally unwelcome, and that is the sensation of pain.

There is a wide range of adjectives to describe feelings of pain, reflecting the different types of pain that can be experienced. Some pains can be described as dull and achy, others sharp and piercing, still others gnawing or stinging. The only common factors between these varying descriptions are that pain is unpleasant, and that the person experiencing the pain would like it to go!

Most people understandably think that when they feel pain there must be something wrong with the bit that is hurting, and this often is the case, of course, in the immediate aftermath of an accident. We stub our toe or sprain an ankle and we feel pain, and most of us will have a fairly good idea of what that particular feeling is like. As the tissues heal, the pain normally subsides and life gets back to normal.

Unfortunately, in some circumstances, the tissues heal but the pain remains. This situation is called *chronic pain*, and it is an area that has undergone a great deal of research in the last fifty years – first by Patrick Wall and Ronald Melzack, who, in the

1970s, developed the 'gate control theory of pain' (subsequently revised by Melzack in 2001 when he developed the 'neuromatrix theory of pain'), and more recently by Australian scientists Professor Lorimer Moseley and David Butler. The latter two researchers, in particular, have contributed significantly to the body of knowledge on pain, and have gone to great lengths to reach mainstream debate with their 'Explain Pain' initiative. This has involved worldwide lecture tours, a widespread online presence and their widely acclaimed eponymous book, all with the intention of helping doctors and manual therapists understand the newly discovered principles underlying chronic pain. The main thrust of their work has been to help people treating musculoskeletal pain to move away from the rather fruitless task of trying to find 'the thing that is wrong in the body', and instead to stand back and look at what is wrong in the individual's overall situation.

THE HEALING PROCESS

The first thing to remember when thinking about chronic pain is the fact that *our bodies heal* – or, to be a little more precise, *adapt*. What should happen, and generally does happen, when we hurt ourselves is that the body lets us know. We experience a level of pain roughly commensurate with the amount of

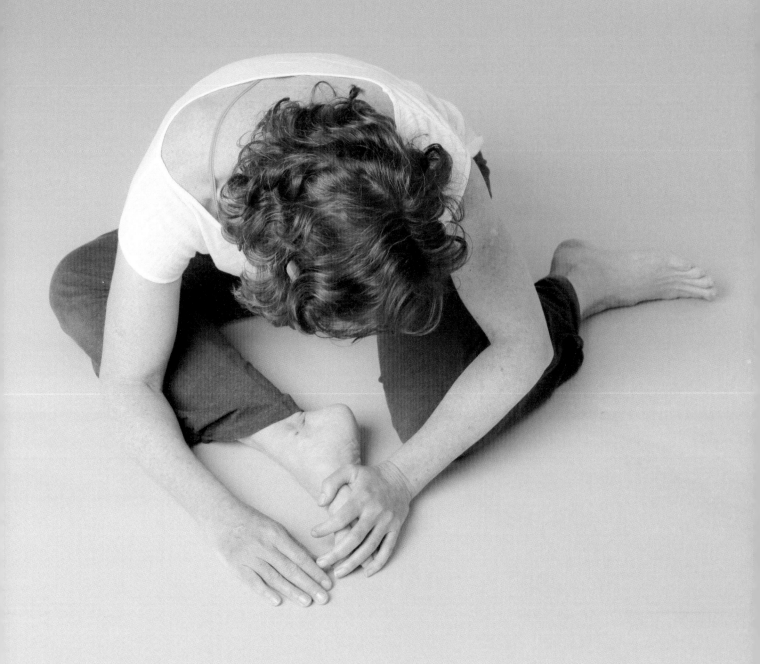

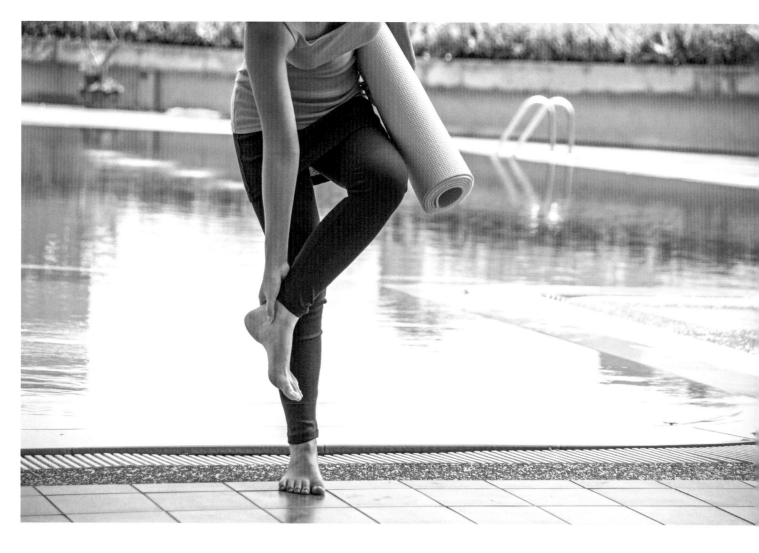

damage we have done to ourselves and, over time, as the body heals as best it can, the pain ebbs away. If it is simply a bumped knee or arm, the pain may subside in a matter of minutes, and the only reminder we are left with is a small bruise. On the other hand, if we snap a tendon it may be severe and it may take weeks for the pain to subside and a few more months before normal function is restored.

If the pain does not subside, however, we need firstly to ask ourselves whether we are doing anything that may be aggravating the injury – something in our everyday life, or maybe even something we are doing in yoga. Sometimes in yoga we can get into the habit of stretching into a pain, thinking we are 'getting to it'. We might describe a 'sweet pain' but often we are simply pulling on a piece of tissue that is already damaged. It may give us temporary relief because it changes the sensory input, but the pain then comes back, and if we keep doing this the injury does not have a chance to heal and may even get worse. Whilst it

is true that we need to keep moving after injury to maintain some range of movement and keep the area 'mapped' in our brain, it is important that we find a balance between the restoration of function and the prevention of re-injury. Remember that after an injury, particularly one that has reduced our activity for some weeks, our tissues – be they ligaments, tendons, muscles or fascia – will have weakened and be less resilient to the movements they are involved in. It will take further weeks of gradual rehabilitation before they are back to normal. A lot of what we have to do here has to do with listening carefully to what we really feel in our body – rather than imposing on it what we think we ought to do – and trying to be patient while our body recovers.

However, it may not be just over-stretching in yoga that is the problem. It may be something intrinsic to the asana. As I discussed in chapter one, certain 'non-functional' yoga asanas can both cause and aggravate injuries if undertaken regularly as, mechanically, there are a few movements that no human body, whatever the type, likes to do. These movements are covered in detail on pages 105–107 of the practice section, but, to summarise here, these are:

- regularly twisting a weight-bearing knee (this might happen in any standing asana that places the back foot at an angle while at the same time squaring the hips up to the front-facing leg – as in the Iyengar-style Warrior I);
- overly compressing the lumbar spine (for instance, in deep back bends such as Scorpion pose (Vrischikasana); and
- shearing actions of the lower lumbar spine (where one vertebra is asked to slide sideways on the vertebra below – such as in the Iyengar-style Triangle, whereby the spine is asked to reach sideways over the leading leg).

Over the years I have seen many injuries that could be attributed to yoga practice, mainly involving knees or lower backs, and memorably including an injury to a colleague whose back 'went' as she strove to reach further sideways in Trikonasana. The number of older teachers I know who have succumbed to the need for knee replacements in their sixties and seventies suggests that their yoga practice may have exacerbated rather than relieved any knee problems.

PAIN AFTER HEALING: BLURRING THE SIGNAL
The second thing we have to bear in mind with pain may seem a little puzzling. It might be that there is no longer any damage to our tissues – they may have healed – yet we are still in pain. This is often the case in long-term or chronic pain, and is a phenomenon that has bewildered physicians throughout history. However, there have been great strides in the last couple of decades in our understanding of how this type of pain comes about.

It used to be thought that nociceptors carried pain signals rather as the optic nerve carries visual signals – in some lay circles nociceptors became known as 'pain nerves' – and that if we damaged ourselves a message would travel up the receptor and ring the pain bell in our brain to let us know we have hurt ourselves, and how bad it is. A moment's reflection will alert us to the fact that this 'damage and signalling' pattern is not necessarily present when it comes to pain, and it is now thought that we do not have nociceptors that act directly like 'pain nerves'. Rather, we have highly modifiable nociception. When we hurt ourselves, nociceptors pass information to the brain from the area of damage, informing it that damage has occurred. However, on the way up to the brain the signal is modified by other parts of the brain. These modifications to the signal will be based on previous experience, on expectation, on one's general state of anxiety and on one's overall sense of well-being (or

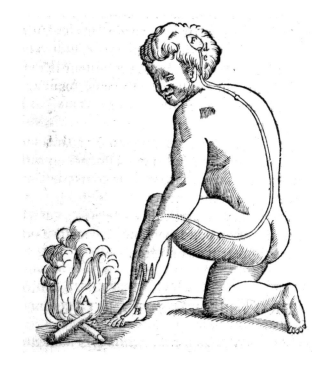

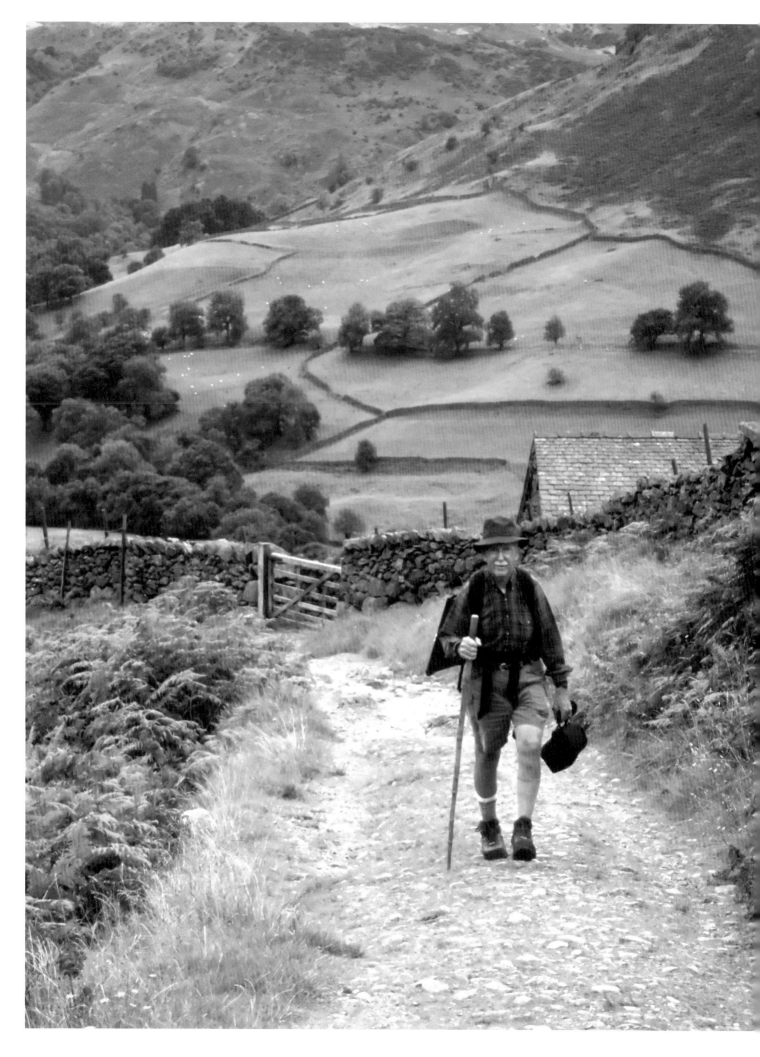

feeling of unease). So, if we stub our toe, something we have probably done many times, the information passed to the brain will be familiar, but it might hurt *more* if we are cold and miserable and *less* so if we are happy and excited. The same information will have been modified by one's current state of mind to either amplify or downscale the sensation.

Some examples of back pain and bad headaches show that severe pain can exist with very little, if any, tissue damage. These seem particularly pointless types of pain, with the signalling being out of proportion to the problem. An extreme example of pain without tissue damage – in fact, without tissue at all – is the extensively studied phenomenon of 'phantom limb' pain, where people who have lost a limb through accident or disease complain of a very particular pain felt 'in' the amputated limb. Conversely, there are times when our attention is absorbed in something and we hurt ourselves but do not really notice until a large bruise appears the next day.

It seems that nociception can be modified in the brain in the following way. Imagine how a person in their forties or fifties with knee or back pain might respond if a health professional tells them that their knee or spinal joints are getting old and worn out. Almost inevitably that person will tend to think it will not get better, that they are simply degenerating. They will adapt and prepare themselves mentally for 'old age' and all the beliefs we have about ageing. This common belief in the link between degeneration and pain may well be driven deeper into our psyche by an X-ray or an MRI scan that depicts the 'damage'. So now any signal we get from a strain in the knee or back will be modified on its journey to the brain by all those worries and anxieties that have lodged in a person's consciousness, and these negative thoughts will 'upregulate' the pain sensation. This is how chronic pain often begins. Our ability to increase or

generate a sense of pain – as well as to ignore and mute pain signals – suggests that the generation of pain is in some ways more akin to emotions than it is to the less changeable external senses such as sight or hearing. The Cartesian view of pain posited that pain represented fairly reliably the severity of damage done to your body and, like the sense of sight, it was a faithful reporter of the situation. The revised view suggests that, like emotions, the feeling of pain can change depending on the situation and expectation.

'Given time, in very many cases the body heals and adapts. We will be left with some physical changes but it will not be accompanied by pain.'

Now, I'm fairly sure that if you are reading this you might well be saying to yourself, 'But surely we know arthritis causes pain, or damaged knee cartilage causes pain, or a disc that has herniated causes pain.' Well, to some extent you are right. When these things first happen, pain and discomfort are often felt. What is less well understood is that, given time, in very many cases the body heals and adapts. We will be left with some physical changes – the disc may still protrude, the cartilage will still show damage and the arthritic joint will show bony change – but it will not be accompanied by pain.

Here are some statistics that might be surprising. In 1994, a paper published in the *New England Journal of Medicine* (NEJM) showed that 52 per cent of asymptomatic subjects had a bulge on at least one level, 27 per cent had a protrusion, and 1 per cent had an extrusion. Thirty-eight per cent had an abnormality of more than one intervertebral disc. The prevalence of bulges, but not of protrusions, increased with age.

In March 2005, a study on knees published in the journal *Osteoarthritis and Cartilage* showed that in forty-four asymptomatic individuals with a mean age of forty-one, twenty-nine had X-ray results of grade 0 (no discernible damage), twelve were grade 1, and three were grade 2. (The scale goes from 0 to 4, with 0 meaning no discernable damage and 4 signifying significant degenerative change.) Five individuals showed evidence of cartilage lesions, with the femoral trochlea, medial femur and patella being those regions most commonly affected. Twelve people (27.3%) showed evidence of osteophytosis ('bone spurs'). Forty-three individuals showed evidence of at least one meniscal abnormality, while twenty-seven individuals (61.4%) had abnormalities in at least three of the four regions of the knee.

A 2004 paper on rotator cuff tears in the *European Journal of Radiology* reported that, from a study of 212 individuals aged between eighteen and eight-three, MRI scans showed that 6 per cent of those between fifty-six and eighty-three had a complete rupture of the supraspinatus tendon, while 40 per cent of those over forty had partial tears of the same muscle. These scans were done on people who had shoulder pain, but, crucially, there were comparative scans of the *other, functional and pain-free shoulder*. This shows that there is a high prevalence of rotator cuff tendon tears in older people that cause no pain and that do not impact on daily activities.

We should not think of things like scoliosis, kyphosis and lordosis as an automatic cause of pain. In fact, it is now fairly well recognised that chronic pain is better correlated with anxiety, depression and worry than it is with more structural conditions like arthritis, disc problems, scoliosis and a host of other 'conditions'. Bodies are remarkably adaptable if they are given time to adapt, and although there are undoubtedly some people who suffer when a condition goes past a point of reorganising itself, there will be many other people with similar conditions who do not have pain. In the last couple

BELOW
MRI scans often unhelpfully increase the perceived link between degeneration and pain.

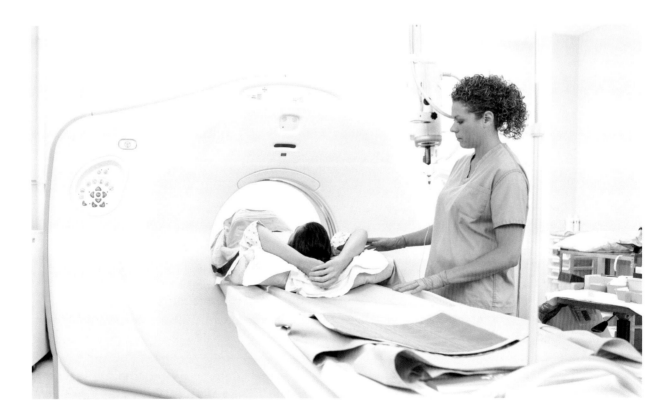

of decades this correlation between structural problems and pain has been dissolving, and better explanations for pain have arisen. We understand better now how the brain modifies nociception based on what we as individuals are led to expect. If our expectations are for a poor outcome, our experience of pain will increase. This is called 'nocebo', the opposite of 'placebo', where our expectations are that things will get better.

EMOTIONAL ELEMENTS IN PAIN

As Suzanne O'Sullivan points out in her wonderful book *It's All in Your Head*, we should not be too surprised by the link between pain and emotions. No one considers blushing a strange phenomenon, after all, but this is a simple example of a bodily response to an emotional situation, as are butterflies in the stomach and tension headaches. Even crying is a somatic response to an emotional or psychological situation. At times in our lives when things are not going well, we notice it in our bodies. We might notice that our heart starts to race and our breathing becomes ragged, our stomach may feel tight and 'uneasy', we may have a headache or develop pain somewhere else in our body. People become unwell and symptoms arise to alert them to the fact that something is not quite right. However, if someone's back starts to hurt or their shoulder seizes up for no apparent reason, we are quick to look for the cause in the body and can get defensive if it is suggested that the problem may be more emotional. But symptoms are not always very clearly related to the problem; in fact, quite often they seem so removed from the cause that we end up treating the symptom rather than the cause. And when the body develops physical symptoms in response to something emotional or psychological, it can all seem rather confusing and unhelpful, particularly if it is implied that the pain is not really there, that we are somehow making it up.

It is true that we may have a genetic or familial tendency to specific physical symptoms, so when things get a bit much we tend to get the symptom

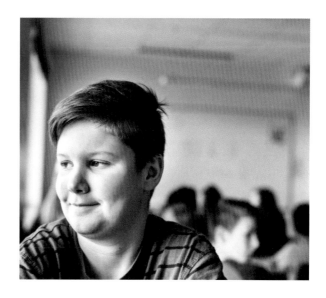

ABOVE
Blushing is a simple example of a bodily response to an emotional situation.

we 'know', be it a skin rash, a tummy upset, back pain or headache. But if we stop and reflect for a moment, we can see that the division of the human being into a mind and a body that are separate and do not affect each other is ridiculous. No 'body' exists without a mind and no 'mind' exists without a body – they form a whole and looking at them separately is a mistake.

Somatisation – the manifestation of psychological distress through bodily symptoms – is well recognised these days (though I dislike the label, which turns a very human response to difficult situations into a condition you can 'have'). So how do we approach situations such as this? As I have argued in the preceding chapters, if we listen more carefully to the sensations and feelings that are generated in our body, and then respond to them as helpfully as we can, we will tend to reduce the sense of inner conflict that gives rise to feelings of disconnect, anxiety, depression and also pain. Ultimately we want to be able to read the signals from our body earlier and earlier, so that we can intervene appropriately before things become too difficult and before more severe symptoms develop.

YOGA PRACTICE, 'NEURO-TAGGING' AND BODY MAPPING

One thing that is very important is that we do not become overly anxious about what injuries and illnesses we are told we 'have'. If it is any of the things described above, or like them in some way, we can be fairly sure that in time the symptoms will pass. In the meantime we should be a little gentler with ourselves, without completely stopping what we are doing.

When it comes to practising yoga asanas, there is something else to bear in mind if we have chronic pain, and that is to not practise with 'distracting' pain, i.e. pain that keeps demanding our attention. This is because of something that has been described by Lorimer Moseley as 'neuro-tagging'. If I move in a particular way and it causes pain, and I keep repeating the same movement regardless, and keep getting the same pain, my brain will begin to associate the two things until it becomes impossible to make the movement without pain, even once the tissues have completely healed. In some cases this 'tagging' becomes extreme until almost any movement hurts and we retreat into immobility, which aggravates the problem further.

If this type of associated pain has developed,

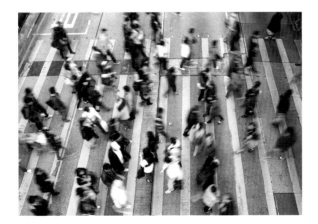

then how do we get out of the situation? Well, there are two or three things that can help and that I try to do with students in pain in my yoga classes. Firstly, we look for a way of undertaking the movement that does not hurt. So, for instance, if rounding the back in a standing forward bend hurts, the student needs to find a way of rounding the back that does not hurt, for example, through experimenting with Cat pose or Child's pose. It is quite common to find that where a standing or seated forward bend gives pain, Cat or Child's pose will not.

It is important to register the fact that it is not just rounding the back that is the problem, but the *context* in which someone rounds their back. In this way the link between the movement and pain can be broken. As the student gains confidence, I normally then try to get them to see how far they can round the back while standing without provoking pain, maybe by softening the knees or putting the hands on the knees to help take the weight – anything to break the link between the two events, rounding the back and pain. It would be similar with knee bending. If bending in one particular situation hurts, I might get them to try it in another situation to gradually nibble away at the association between the pain and the movement. It is also useful to get them to pay attention to other sensations during the movement – the body's contact with the floor, for instance, or feelings of softening or stiffening in the body, or the sensation of the breath and the shifting of weight as we move. All these things will help people to gradually move away from mentally 'going' to their pain and help them to experience themselves in a more comfortable way.

Another important thing to consider when dealing with chronic pain is the issue of 'mapping', which I have discussed in the preceding chapters. There is some evidence to support the theory that chronic pain is associated with bodies that are poorly mapped. It also seems to be the case that chronic pain causes a 'smudging' of the injured part of our body's representation in the brain. It seems that when we injure ourselves, neurons that are adjacent to the area of the brain that represents the injured part are recruited into the map to highlight

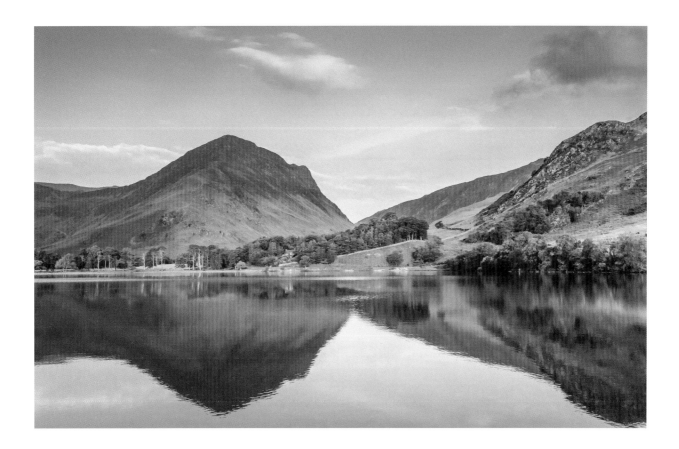

what has happened, so we can 'feel it' more. This is appropriate, and as we recover, those recruited neurons should go back to resuming their normal duties. If, however, we become anxious about the injury, if we stop moving it, and if we give it too much worrisome attention, then those neurons, instead of resuming normal duties, may recruit even more neurons to assist the area we are protecting. Soon the 'brain map' of the damaged area will have expanded beyond its normal boundaries. This is called 'neuro-smudging', a term coined by David Butler, and it is associated with changes in sensation and chronic pain.

When it comes to body mapping and pain, yoga can help in three main ways. Firstly, it can reduce anxiety about the pain for all the reasons stated above, perhaps predominantly by demonstrating that after some weeks it is very unlikely that there is still tissue damage. Secondly, it can help redefine the 'brain map' of the damaged area by putting the area through attentive and varying movements and, as confidence increases, gradually increasing the range of movement until it is back to normal function. And thirdly, we can help people grade their exposure to the movements that hurt them by slowing their movements down and helping them notice at what point things become worrying for them, and then, allowing them to ease towards and away from the movement until they develop some confidence and can increase their range of movement.

Yoga teachers and practitioners are extremely well placed to address musculoskeletal problems and pain as long as we understand some basic principles: that we should not put the body through movements it is not well evolved to deal with; that we should not force movements in an attempt to 'get somewhere'; that we should practise with attentive curiosity rather than with fear and anxiety; and that we should nurture within us and within our classes the notion that persistent, regular, sensible movements will, over time, allow the body to adapt, either structurally or neurologically, until any symptoms and feelings of pain fade away.

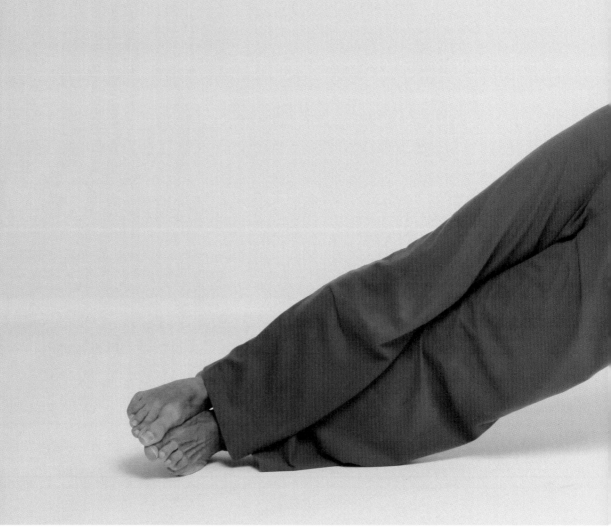

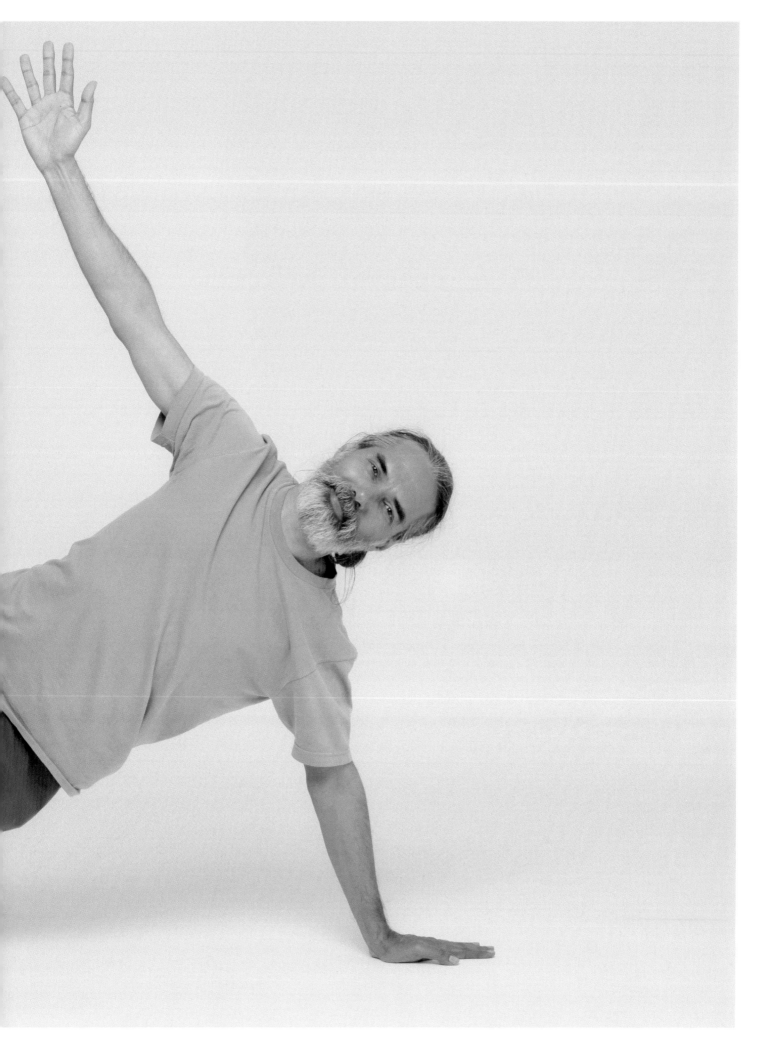

FIVE

YOGA BEYOND THE MAT

A humanist perspective

Yoga holds a unique place in the exploration of the human condition. On the one hand, it can draw on a rich historical heritage, while on the other, the direct experience of the practitioner keeps it forever in the present.

Having a history is useful, as I pointed out in chapter one of this book, as it gives context to the modern practice of yoga – or at least it has the potential to do so. There is also a danger, though, of coming to be led by yoga's heritage, so that instead of seeking to build on the understandings of those who have gone before, we conform our experience to fit what we have been led to expect. This, I would argue, is the biggest challenge to the modern yogi.

So what are the advances and values of the modern world, and how do they fit with yoga? In this chapter, I will attempt to outline some of the discoveries and insights that have made an impact on me and enriched my understanding of the human condition and, consequently, of yoga, which is much more than simply a series of physical postures. In fact, a core element of yoga practice is about subjective noticing, tuning in to how we feel and responding appropriately. This is the most basic act of self-regulation.

First of all it is worth reflecting on the most difficult problem we face as human beings: that we know we are going to die, a knowledge that (almost certainly) no other species has to live with. A starting point that stresses that we are born alone and that we die alone – and that we do not carry on after that – might appear pretty bleak, but for me this is the bottom line. I believe that facing up to this reality is the ultimate challenge of being human, and I do not want to fabricate any false promises or positions to try to make myself feel better about the situation. Rather, I want to develop the qualities that enable me to live a life with this knowledge and without fear.

Coming to terms with the concept of dying and being alone is essential, and much of our existence is inevitably spent dealing with this recognition, whether consciously or unconsciously. If acknowledged consciously, this existential challenge may inspire us to live our lives as richly as we can, knowing that our time here is brief. It may help us fathom meaning in the way we live our lives, and help us not to waste time on the superficial inanities that surround us in the modern world. Conversely, if it goes unacknowledged, we may find that a nagging, subconscious worry about dying or losing someone we love drives us into various distractions that take our mind off the dilemma – distractions that can only succeed for so long, as the inevitable moves ever closer.

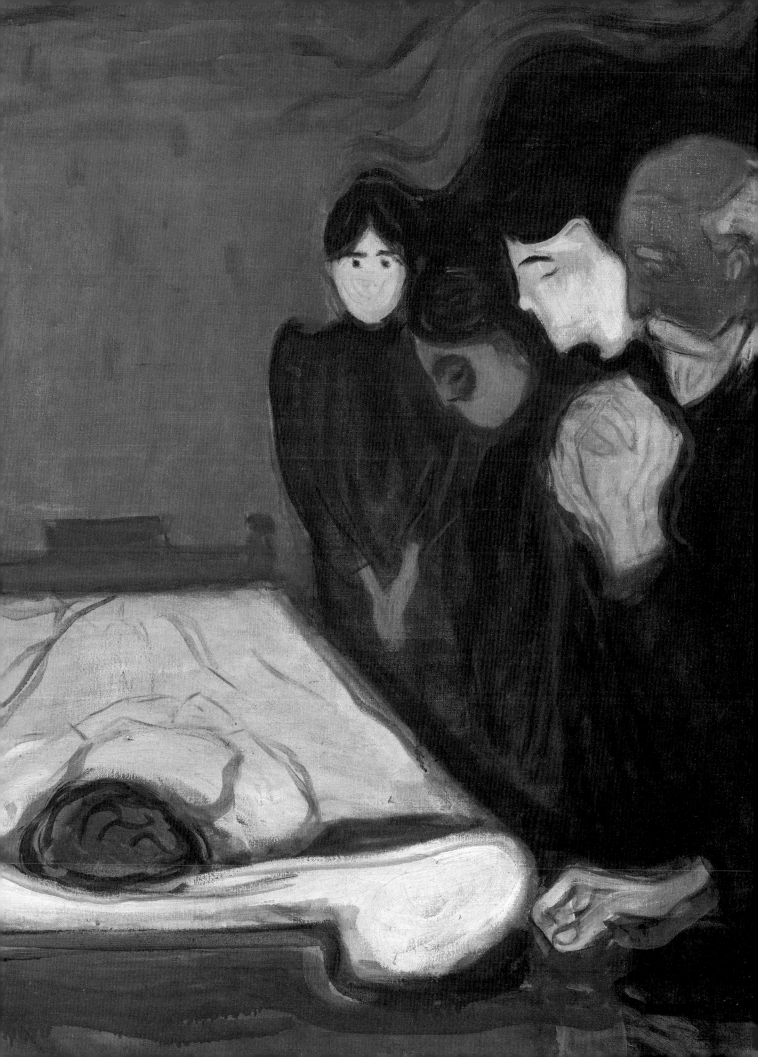

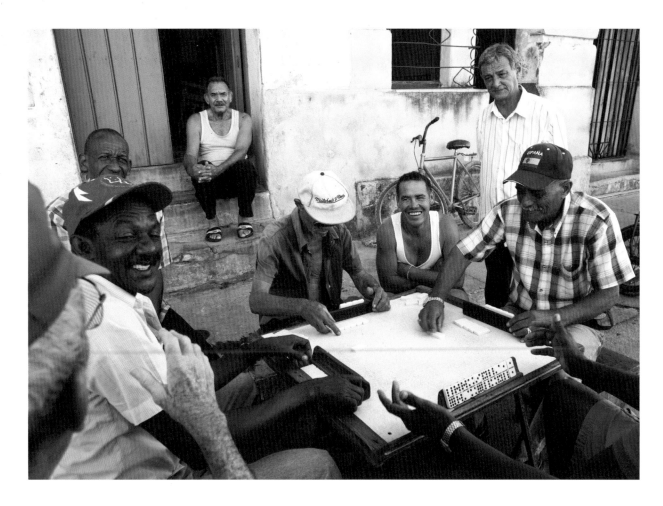

ABOVE
Human beings are a social species, and the quailty of our relationships impacts deeply on our state of well-being.

So where do we look for consolation for this age-old problem? One key place to start is to look to our innately social nature as human beings. Good relationships are a powerful balm for coping with feelings of uncertainty and isolation, and without relationships we fail to thrive. Very young children will die without human contact, even when they are fed and watered. A slightly older child will suffer brain damage if human contact is removed or reduced to subsistence levels. Throughout our lives the quality of the relationships we form impacts deeply on our state of well-being. Because we are a social species, we thrive in communities – and conversely, being separated from our fellow humans causes us to suffer. To isolate someone is one of the worst punishments we can inflict on them.

Loneliness is the discomforting feeling that arises

when our relationships and communities are not up to the mark. We need to heed this feeling, as our feelings are our primary means of social and personal self-regulation. Though it is evident that people have differing needs for social contact, it is very unusual for a person to thrive in isolation (something examined by John T. Cacioppo in his book *Loneliness: Human Nature and the Need for Social Connection*). Being a hermit is almost certainly not the right aspiration for good human health, even if most of us feel the need to be alone from time to time.

We stop 'aloneness' becoming loneliness through our ability to form relationships. The skill with which we do this will go a very long way in determining whether our lives are happy or not. It is not too difficult to extrapolate from this that moral frameworks evolve out of social frameworks. In our search for better relationships and the avoidance of isolation we need to look after those who would look after us – we will scratch their back if they scratch ours. As societies grow in complexity, so do our skills in social interaction, and the richness in our emotional responses to the world.

It is now well established that all mammals are capable of at least four basic emotions, namely fear, anger/rage, distress/panic at separation from a parent or group, and an urge to seek and explore. All animals have dedicated neural circuits for these emotions, as Jaak Panksepp documented in his book *Affective Neuroscience: The Foundations of Human and Animal Emotions*. 'Higher' emotions are less easy to determine, and whether other animals feel empathy, envy or schadenfreude is uncertain – but it is probably a question of a sliding scale. A hedgehog might not experience such feelings, whereas the great apes almost certainly do. Human beings, as we well know, have a complex repertoire of overlapping emotions, each with a particular felt sense that alerts us to their presence.

Of course, it is increasingly recognised that our relationships do not exist in a vacuum. We live in a complex world in which we are embedded. The theory of evolution demonstrates that there is a process of co-creation that goes on between all living things and their environment. We are shaped by our surroundings, and we shape the environment we are in, and to flourish in this world it is wise to pay good attention to this relationship. The consequences of an exploitative relationship can be witnessed all around us, most depressingly in climate change, the depletion of the earth's biodiversity and the suffering of animals for commercial gain.

YOGA, SELF-EXPLORATION AND PAYING ATTENTION

So what has all this got to do with yoga? From my perspective, it has everything to do with yoga. Our yoga practice, if performed intelligently, is an extremely useful method of self-exploration. Through it we learn about the way in which we inhabit our bodies, we learn about muscular habits and patterns that we have laid down in our life, and we start to find out what these patterns mean. We also notice the emotional patterns we have laid down over a lifetime, and our tell-tale 'feeling signature'.

'Our yoga practice, if performed intelligently, is an extremely useful method of self-exploration.'

I think most of us would agree that, at least on some level, we are seeking a life that is nourishing and rewarding. Whether that is what we have is a different question. If our life does not seem that way, how is it that we arrived at an unintended destination? It seems to me that old habits and unhelpful emotional maps might have something to do with it.

It has been said that by the time you are forty, you have the face you deserve. To some extent our bodies are 'set' in a similar way, although I would not use the word 'deserve'. Rather, our bodies represent the lives we have lived thus far, our history and our emotional responses to our experiences.

Many of the habits that our nervous systems have developed – habits exhibited by our muscles and our emotions – reflect the struggles we have encountered and survived as children. They represent the defences and bracings we have needed to get through life. We shut down difficult feelings by holding ourselves in a particular way, in an attempt to make ourselves feel safe. Our diaphragm, shoulders and hip flexors all play major roles in the containment of feelings, but any muscles can participate. This is particularly true when we try to hide our discomfort. The muscular 'disguises' we wear to avoid revealing our real feelings eventually become familiar and part of us.

Emotional and physical habits get played out over and over again in everyday life and often bring us discomfort or pain. Therapists might be able to help with the identification of our physical and emotional problems but the real work starts when we begin to self-reflect on our habits and patterns, to discover ourselves and slowly strip away a mantle we no longer need. What is really significant to notice is that it is not about trying to reveal the pearl that exists somewhere in the mythical core of our being. Rather it is about understanding that it is the conduct of the relationship we have with people and things that is significant. If we are suffering, whether physically or emotionally, it can feel easier to blame something or someone for our discomfort. We can blame a muscle – 'I have a psoas spasm' – as if that muscle had a life of its own, disconnected from the rest of us. Or we can blame our wife or husband for being unreasonable – again, as if their behaviour were separate from our responses to them. Most difficulties in life lie in the relationship between things rather than in the things themselves.

Once we manage to remove our unnecessary reflex responses to life, we discover that we have choices in the way we respond. Instead of doing what we have always done, we can do something different, and our relationship to our body or to a person can become more useful. What we are actually doing here is re-mapping our relationship to things, making new and enriching connections in the neurons of our brain, enabling ourselves to change our behaviour. As other options appear, we become freer. We are better off than if we plod along a reflex pathway that is self-confining.

It is not easy to move away from old ingrained ways of being, but it starts in yoga practice with the gradually improving capacity to pay attention. Initially this might simply be noticing how we organise the body in space – noticing, for example, whether our feet are well organised or not. It can soon develop into an awareness of muscular movement patterns, of how we deal with breathing and, perhaps later, how we respond to a certain person who perhaps makes us feel emotionally defensive.

Slowly we can find out more about ourselves, and by doing so become better able to choose our responses, thus improving our relationships. This, I think, defines maturity. As we get older and lose the spring of youth, the sense of being a more complete person is good compensation. Friendships can broaden and deepen, and our capacity to love

– the pinnacle of human achievement – becomes greater. And so the life we live, the only life we have, becomes richer and more nourishing.

Those people who are interested in this kind of personal journey can suffer a fair amount of discomfort on the way, just as taking off familiar old clothes can leave us feeling vulnerable or bereft. But as we put better strategies in place, our life can take on a new and rewarding depth.

LOVE, RELATIONSHIPS AND DEVELOPMENT

Knowing where our difficulties start is intriguing and can be useful to examine. Emerging research in neuroscience suggests, perhaps unsurprisingly, that these problems start to develop early in our life, in the context of our relationship with our parents. The wonderfully revealing book by Sue Gerhardt called *Why Love Matters: How Affection Shapes a Baby's Brain* shows the effects of parental love on brain development. Our current understanding goes something like this: when a baby is born it is completely unable to deal with or regulate its feelings. When discomfort develops in a child up to the age of about three, the child experiences stress. We can now measure levels of stress in babies by swabbing their mouths and measuring their levels of the 'stress hormone' cortisol. As Gerhardt asserts:

> Human babies are born with the expectation of having stress managed for them. They tend to have low levels of cortisol in the first few months, as long as caring adults maintain their equilibrium through touch, stroking, feeding and rocking. But their immature systems are also very unstable and reactive; they can be plunged into very high cortisol levels if there is no one to respond to them. Babies cannot manage their own cortisol.

She goes on to note that stress in infancy, such as consistently being ignored when you cry, is particularly hazardous because high levels of cortisol in the early months of life can also affect the development of other neurotransmitter systems whose pathways are still being established:

They are still immature and are not fully developed even by weaning time. Babies of withdrawn mothers, for example, have lower epinephrine, norepinephrine and dopamine than other babies. When stressed, these various biochemical systems may become skewed in ways that make it more difficult for the individual to regulate his or her feelings later in life.

For many parents, the information revealed in Gerhardt's book makes for uncomfortable reading. I for one was brought up in a time when being left to cry was considered to be good for a baby's lungs. Mothers were told to feed their babies every four hours. We are now starting to learn that these ideas are wrong. They may have been well meant but they caused suffering. On reflection, we can see, too, that such approaches are counter-intuitive. Mothers and fathers are 'wired' to respond to a crying baby, not to ignore it.

The reason some parents manage better than others almost certainly has something to do with their own childhoods, and how well regulated they were as babies. A child unable to regulate his or her feelings will grow into an adult (and possibly parent) who struggles with those same feelings. They may also find it almost impossible to engage with their own baby's emotions in a productive and responsive way, and so the cycle continues.

I feel that we are now approaching a time when this negative cycle can be broken, and we may eventually be able to produce generations of children who are more 'in touch' with their feelings. This will mean that as adults they will not have to look to

BELOW
No other species has such a long period of parental depency as that of humans.

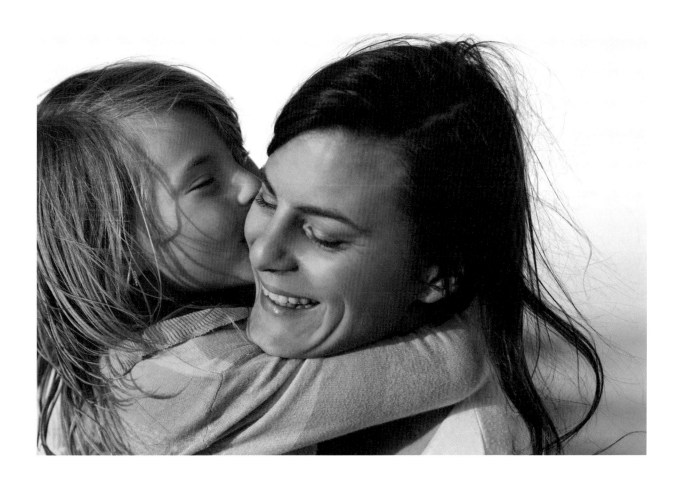

other people or belief systems to do their regulating for them, beyond providing a healthy level of emotional and social support.

Gerhardt, whose work echoes John Bowlby's attachment theory, believes that the problems individuals encounter in adult relationships are often rooted in the poorly developed relationships they had with their parents as children. If we are to make progress in the arena of relationships, we need to practise improving our responses to situations. Shouting at a child who is hungry or tired and making his/her frustrations known is not just unhelpful, but also confusing for the child, affecting how he or she learns to relate to and express physical and emotional feelings.

No other species on the planet has such a long period of parental dependency as that of humans. For several years, we need adult members of the society to help us survive. If an older person says to a child in an authoritative voice, 'Do not play with snakes,' the child will tend to obey. Evolution will weed out the rashly experimental child. 'Poke it and see' is not a good survival strategy where snakes are concerned. It is seemingly inbred in humans to do what authority figures tell us. And if we have been psychologically primed by an absent or emotionally neglectful parent to continue to search for what we missed in childhood, and a charismatic guru or religious teacher comes along, our past can then drive us into a predictable relationship with this new parental figure. Sadly, the childlike trust that we have in such figures can lead to the development of

BELOW
A sea anemone will open up to the world when its circumstances are right and safe.

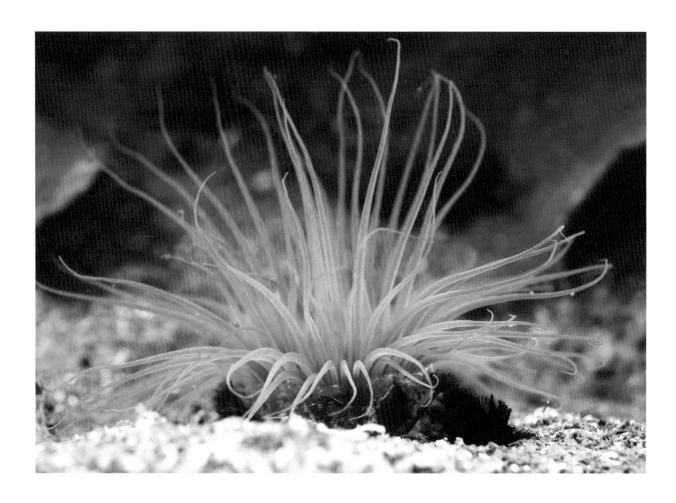

abusive relationships between the teacher/authority figure and the student, and as I write these words in 2017 both the yoga world and the world at large are being rocked by stories of abuse by the powerful of those in subordinate positions.

There are, of course, many shades of grey in the way the past drives our present. We all know that feeling of repeating old mistakes over and over again or, in a bodily sense, getting that same headache, stomach ache or backache in the same circumstances. It is clear that in some way our history has set us up for these patterns of behaviour, and that they are very difficult to resist. Many people have made a lot of money playing on this knowledge. So many self-help books tell us that living in the present will solve our problems, and to a certain extent they are correct: if you can free yourself of your past, you free yourself of your patterning. But one cannot simply will this to happen.

YOGA AND THE 'PROTO SELF'

It can be informative to understand how emotions are formed in the brain. As it turns out, the body is heavily involved. Neurobiologist Antonio Damasio is one of the world's leading researchers into consciousness and the emergence of feelings and emotions. He argues, in his book *The Feeling of What Happens: Body and Emotion in the Making of Conciousness*, that consciousness arrives out of a pre-set condition he calls 'the proto self' – a kind of default condition of the human organism, one that is mapped in the lower centres of the brain. It is important to recognise that we are not conscious of the proto self, but it is the foundation on which all consciousness rests. The next level of consciousness arises when any part of our sensory nervous system is activated. Any input creates a change in the proto self, which responds to all stimuli.

It is the change or modification of the proto self which makes us aware we exist. It seems to be the case that we know we have a self because we are constantly stimulating the proto self with a stream of sensory input. This input may be external, a sound or smell, or it may be internal, such as thirst

or tension. There is never a waking moment when the proto self is not being modified, and so we are constantly aware of our existence. When we sleep and have no input we do not know we exist.

Damasio calls this level of consciousness the 'core self'. It provides, he argues, the basis for the next level of consciousness, 'the autobiographical self'. We are all familiar with our autobiographical self, formed of the memories we recall, which allow us to feel a connection to our childhood even though every molecule of our body will have changed since that time.

However, memories are distinct from feelings, and feelings, says Damasio, are the substrate for emotions:

Punishment causes organisms to close themselves in, freezing and withdrawing from their surroundings. Reward causes organisms to open themselves up and out towards their environment, approaching it, searching it, and by doing so increasing both their opportunity for survival and their vulnerability. This fundamental duality is apparent in a creature as simple as a sea anemone. Its organism, devoid of brain and equipped only with a simple nervous system, is little more than a gut with two openings, animated by two sets of muscles, some circular others lengthwise. The circumstances surrounding the sea anemone determine what its entire organism does: open up to the world like a blossoming flower – at which point water and nutrients enter its body and supply it with energy – or close itself in a contracted flat pack, small, withdrawn, nearly imperceptible to others. The essence of joy and sadness, of approach and avoidance, of vulnerability and safety, are as apparent in this simple dichotomy of brainless behaviour as they are in the mercurial emotional changes of a child at play.

There is a peculiar division that Damasio makes with regard to feelings and emotions. He believes that emotions precede feelings, that our response to events occurs before the feelings arise. In fact, he argues, it is the response that causes the feelings.

So when something joyful occurs, we respond; we smile, we breathe differently, we relax our shoulders, and this causes the feeling of joy. In other words, it is the change in the physical infrastructure that allows the feelings to arise. Although this view has come under criticism from Jaak Panksepp, who argues in the book *Affective Neuroscience* that feelings are hard-wired in regions of the brain, he also concedes that bodily states reinforce feeling states even if they are not the progenitors of them. Either

'We all have emotional "default" settings, but with no particular remembered event to cause such feelings.'

way, the relationship between emotions and bodies seems to be an intimate one, and one that most people will already have some sense of.

It is often said that it is hard to be sad if you put on a smile. It is harder still if you normalise your breathing and adopt a relaxed body posture. Such experiments reveal an intimate relationship between the state of our body and how we feel. It is not a big leap of reasoning to recognise that our habitual patterns of muscular tension will be associated with habitual patterns of feeling and thinking. It is very difficult to free ourselves from repeating cycles of discomfort, emotional or physical, if we carry our past around in unrecognised muscular patterns.

Internally, all kinds of homeostatic mechanisms ensure that our bodies continue to function. Emotions are our external regulators and we have developed a rich set of these to regulate the relationships that exist in social groups. In more primitive social structures, such as those of apes and monkeys, emotions are probably less sophisticated than those of human beings, but it is easy to see how displays of emotion keep the groups in some

sort of order. Mutual fear of predators encourages cooperative feelings, anger and fear establish pecking orders, and so on. Any individual ignoring the signals risks violence from stronger males, or expulsion from the group.

Ignoring powerful feelings for too long can, it seems, throw out the feedback mechanisms for our internal regulators. Cortisol levels rise and the risk of illness is increased. Equilibrium – and good health – demands that we respond to feelings and emotions.

However, identifying a feeling or emotion before acting upon it appropriately is not as easy as it seems. Many feelings are vague, held as they are by patterns of responding that originate deep in our individual self. Commonly we have emotional 'default' settings – we might be angry, ebullient, or melancholic people – but with no particular remembered event to cause such feelings. In such people, small triggers might initiate a cascade of emotional responses. They may, indeed, wonder why they respond so powerfully to certain events. Anyone who has had a relationship with such a person will recognise how difficult it can be. On some level you recognise you are dealing with someone who has lost any choice in how they respond to a particular stimulus. Ultimately, these relationships can become unsatisfactory, lacking as they do spontaneity, depth and surprise.

Through yoga practice we can discover how we tighten our jaw and neck, or fix our diaphragm, and with time we can lose this old and unnecessary tension. The more often we practise without the pattern, the weaker the pattern becomes. And so life becomes simpler. In the bigger picture, this has significant implications – the type of yoga practice I am talking about can lead to greater self-knowledge in all aspects of our lives.

RIGHT
Picasso's 'Melancholy Woman' (1902).

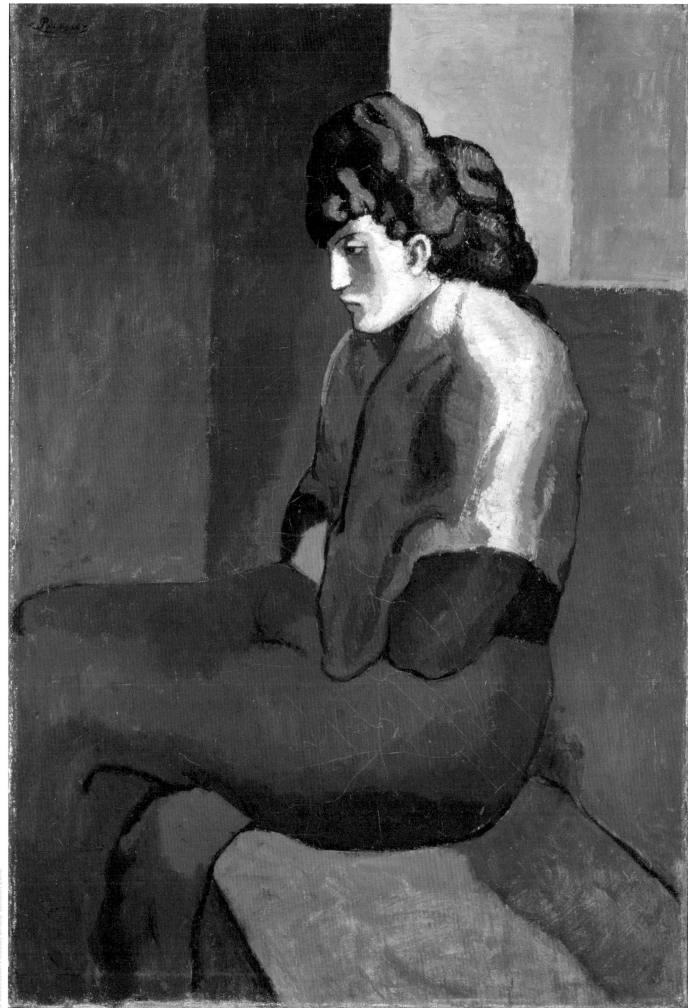

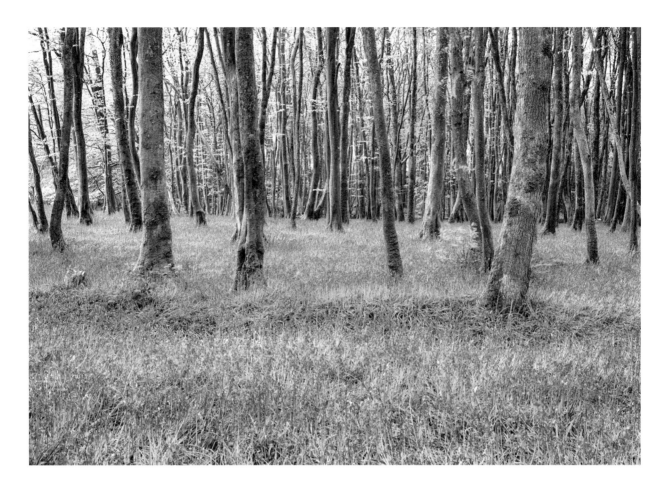

The natural world can nourish
us at the deepest level.

Understanding ourselves better leads in turn to greater self-trust. There is nothing that interferes with good relationships more than a lack of self-trust. When we do not trust ourselves, we have to put our trust in other people, and so our own identity slowly becomes dissipated. We become less attractive to some people, with whom we lose contact, and more controlled by others.

Yoga brings into question how we learn, particularly from our teachers; or if we are teachers, how we teach. If we are interested in developing 'whole' people, people who can trust themselves and make intelligent choices in life, we need to make sure the conditions are right to bring about such an outcome. We need to consider how we establish an environment where self-trust develops.

Learning environments must feel safe. Students need to be able to ask questions without feeling intimidated. Although yoga classes require introspection and peacefulness, they are also likely to provoke questioning. Discussion and debate engages people in a way that 'top-down' teaching

cannot. It breaks down dogma and reduces the tendency for any 'teacher worship' to develop. It also fosters social interaction, something that can be helpful in yoga and life generally.

The larger part of this book explains the neurology and physiology relevant to yoga practice. I have argued that we need some understanding of the biomechanics of the body to avoid injury, and I have tried to explain that the breath needs to be responsive rather than controlled. I have asserted, too, that some ways of engaging with the body are better than others. I hope I have expressed these points in a way that readers can follow, but I welcome disagreement and debate.

Not all yoga is like this. There is a long-standing tradition in yoga that wisdom is passed down from guru to student, and because much of yoga's

'There are times when uncertainty can feel frustrating, but it is one of the conditions of reason. There is no all-knowing position to be had.'

history has been dominated by mysticism (i.e. the perception that insight can be attained through dedicated practice), there has long been a tendency for obscuring knowledge. The serious yoga student will, at some point, have to make a decision about belief – namely, whether to abandon one's critical faculties and perception of the world and to pursue a belief that makes some big promises, a world where suffering can be transcended, where even death may be an illusion, as reflected in the ideas of karma, *samskara* and rebirth that permeate Hindu thought. In many cases this involves surrendering to a guru. This contrasts starkly with self-trust and the idea of developing choice and reason. In fact, belief and reason are very different and can lead us in very different directions.

I can understand the relief that surrendering to a belief might bring, but it has a cost – the loss of the ability to question and to be open to new ideas. Belief systems cannot stand scrutiny; you buy into the belief or you stand outside it. It is almost impossible to half-believe. In belief systems, doubt is seen as an obstacle to the truth.

In a system based on rational thought, questions and doubts are assets, providing fuel for debate and discovery. There are times when uncertainty can feel frustrating, but it is one of the conditions of reason. We do not know everything and there is no all-knowing position to be had.

What do we risk losing if we decide not to believe? Not much, I think. A simple human life is not an arid one. Anyone who has experienced the ecstasy of falling in love, the breathtaking beauty of nature, the wonder of music and art, and the curiosity engendered by self-exploration, knows that the world can nourish us at the deepest level. The knowledge that my molecules were formed in stars, and that my family line forms an unbroken chain through hundreds of millions of years back to the primordial soup, makes the hairs on the back of my neck stand on end. This and the good friendships we form in life enhance our lives and us as individuals.

The needs of society today are different from those of the society that gave birth to yoga. The idea of rigid duty and unwavering faith in God are no longer as widely appealing as they once were. Some may ask how we regulate social behaviour and hone our moral and ethical principles if we have moved away from the frameworks that gave life structure in the past. Many books have been written on this subject and this is not one of them. However, I am an optimist and if I believe in anything, I believe in humanity.

The world is shaped by individuals. The more clearly we understand ourselves and our motivations, the more chance we have of acting well in the world, and this is really my main focus. Yoga can help us to act with understanding and self-awareness, to become mature in the full sense of the word. It is a positive force in a world that struggles to accommodate change.

BELOW
Everything in the world is interconnected; our molecules were originally formed in stars.

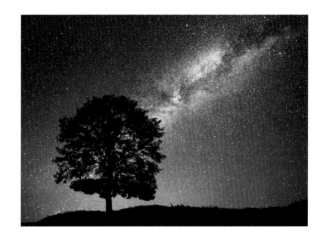

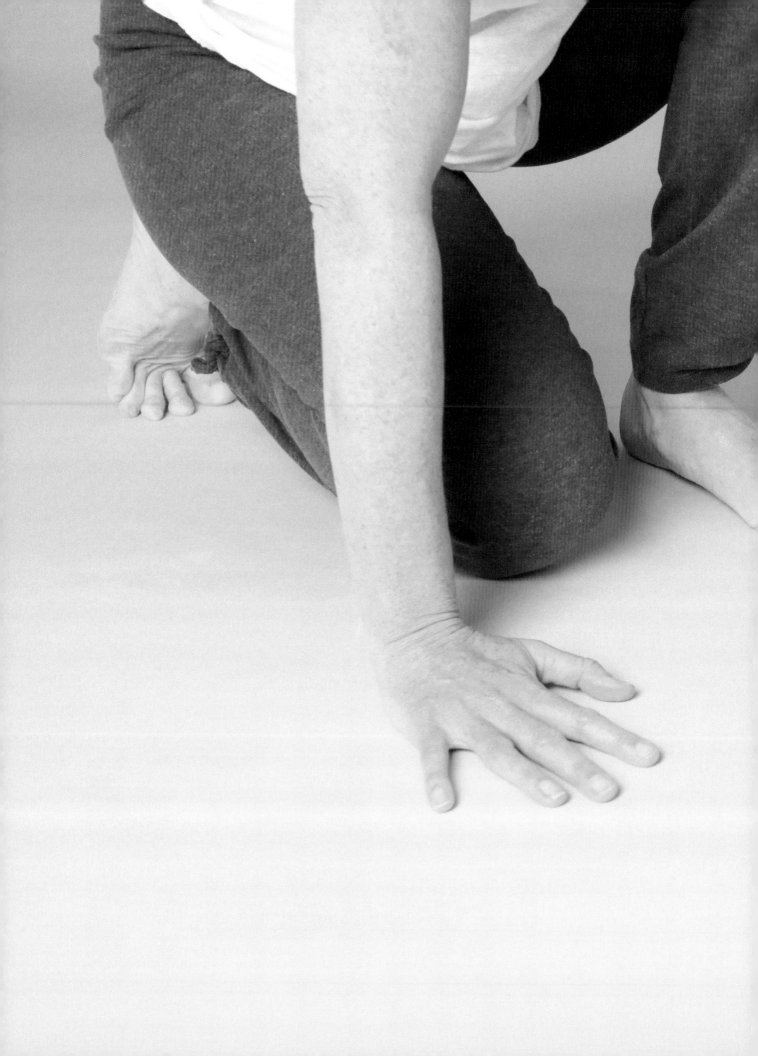

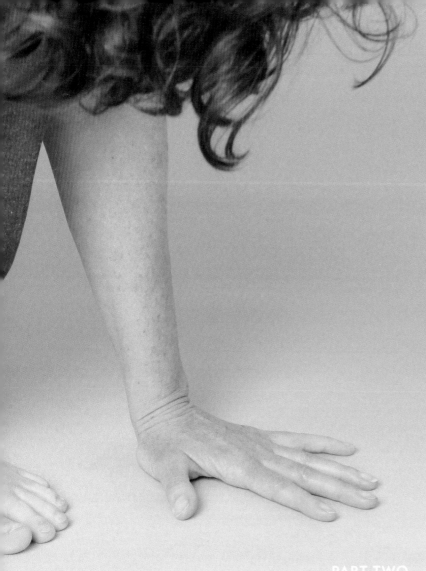

PART TWO

THE PRACTICE

—— SIX ——

APPROACHING OUR PRACTICE

Why we need to stop thinking of yoga as exercise

Exercise, in the gym sense of the word, tends to have three main impacts on the body, depending on the type of exercise undertaken. These are strengthening muscles, improving range of movement and increasing aerobic capacity. As ends in themselves, none of these aspects of exercise have any significant lasting benefit to the individual. We all, of course, benefit from an active lifestyle, where activity is part of our daily lives (whether it's manual work, regular dog walking or cycling some distance to work every day). But if exercise is simply a discipline that is grudgingly tacked on to some point of the day, the benefits will be transient. This is because exercise, in this sense of the word, focuses on our bodily *structure*, and the goal here is generally to make changes on that level. Yoga, on the other hand, is particularly useful for making changes on the *neurological* level. Though these two things are clearly not separate, our *intention* will influence the approach we take when we practise yoga.

We tend to go harder at things if we are trying to change structure – lift more weights… run a bit further… stretch that little bit more. Because, with exercise, that is how improvement comes. If, on the other hand, we are trying to influence the nervous system, we will tend to take a more nuanced approach, because now the intention is something to do with discrimination – how we discriminate this feeling from that, how our breath changes when we do something, or how much effort we are putting into any movement. To notice these sorts of things, we may need to slow a movement down, do a smaller movement and repeat it to see if we can discriminate further. These types of changes persist, as once we have noticed something, it is difficult to un-notice it – a very different approach to simple 'exercise', as many of us know it.

There is another important point: if we stop exercising, the gains we have made to structure will be lost in about eight weeks and we will then have to start again. However, learning to pay attention with/to the nervous system is something that easily comes off the mat; we can apply the approach to almost everything we do until we feel we have really embodied our yoga. For example, when going for a straightforward walk, you may start to become aware that as you are able to relax a little more, the arms and shoulders swing more freely, the rib cage rotates a little and the pelvis starts to move more. This all gives our walking a sense of ease because the whole body becomes involved in the process of walking rather than just the legs.

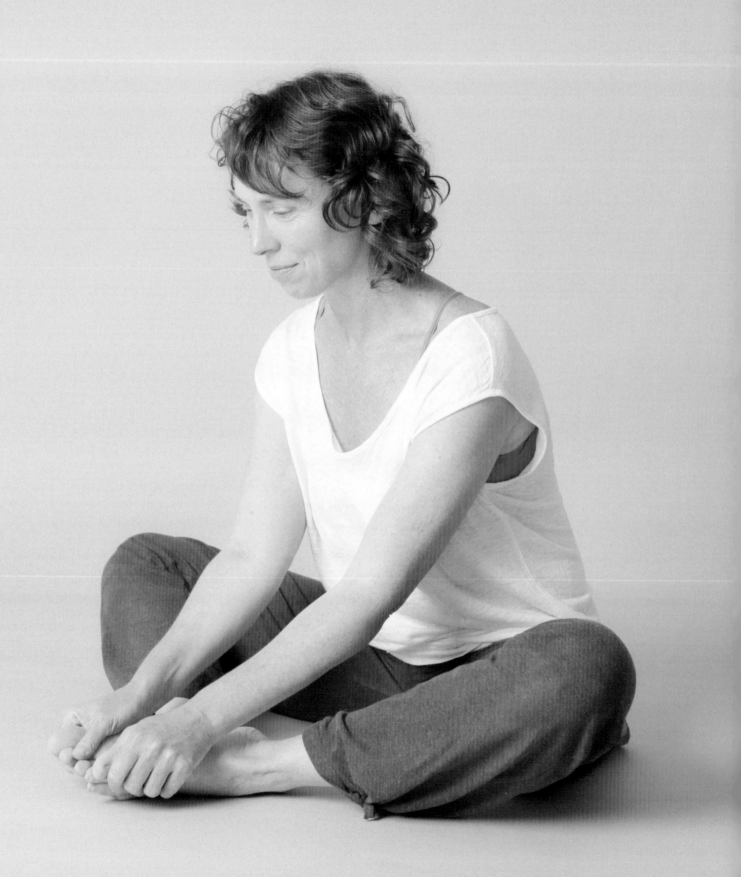

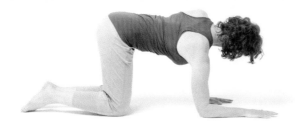

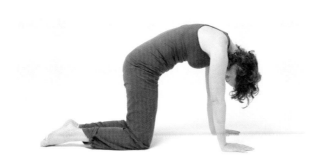

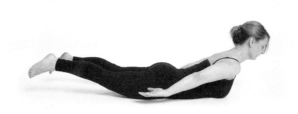

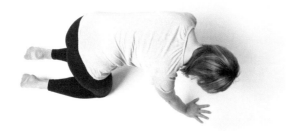

ABOVE
A key aspect of yoga practice is to maintain, or restore, normal human movement. This means asking the spine to turn, flex, extend and side bend, to some extent.

MOVEMENT AND SENSE OF SPACE

So, if we are not exercising when we practise yoga in this way, what are we doing? Well, perhaps the most structural aspect of practice is simply practical, and that is to either maintain, or try to restore, 'normal human movement', as outlined in chapter one of this book. This involves putting our spine, hips, shoulders, feet and ankles through movements that an active person would require to meet their everyday needs.

Briefly, this would involve movements that ask the spine to flex, turn, side bend and extend to some extent. The hips, knees and feet need to be able to allow you to get up and down from the floor with ease, and also give you the freedom to be able to sit on the floor comfortably, preferably in at least two different positions. The arms and shoulders need to be able to reach up and also reach behind our back.

However, optimal health requires more than this. In particular, it requires us to have an accurate sense of proprioception i.e. where our bodies are in space. Our sense of proprioception develops through exploratory movements, and improves rapidly if there is a clear intention behind the exploration. Think of a child learning to feed itself, or a learner driver getting the 'feel' of where the mirror, handbrake and pedals are in a car. These movements are initially clumsy but improve with the reward of steady progress. As such, it is useful to be clear about our intention for whatever it is we are practising. It may simply be the intention to stabilise the foot in a standing balance, or the quality of smoothness or flow as you move from one position to another.

When we move less, when we are sedentary in our lives, the proprioceptive sense of ourselves becomes poorly distinguished. This becomes very apparent when we notice the difference between the way we can move our hands and our feet. Modern life asks very little of the feet, and it shows: very few people have any dexterity when it comes to moving feet and toes (which is why I often start my yoga practice and classes with movements to address this, as described in the box on the far right, 'Find your feet'). However, those people born without arms are almost as skillful with their feet as their able-bodied counterparts are with their hands.

Apart from the obvious benefits of being able to move with skill, people who have well-mapped movements seem to be less prone to developing chronic pain, as I explored in chapter four. In fact, Australian-born pain researcher David Butler – co-author, with Lorimer Moseley, of *Explain Pain* (2013) – argues that pain itself causes a degrading of our body map and one of the strategies to recover from chronic pain is to practise movements that help us re-notice ourselves.

NOTICING EFFORT AND TRANSITIONS

Another useful thing to focus on is the amount of effort we put into our movements. Our nervous systems developed under evolutionary pressure, and efficiency of action was paramount for survival. We would have needed to move as skillfully and effectively as possible to survive, so there would have been no wasteful expenditure of energy. In modern times, where there is no survival pressure driving our movements, we tend to stop improving them when they are sufficiently good to accomplish our needs. But this is often far from the optimal situation (optimal being the ability to move and carry out tasks with minimum expenditure of effort). It is helpful, then, to consider optimal movement when we practise, and to listen closely to our bodies to notice any undue effort we might be expending.

In this regard, we need to be particularly alert to any 'transitions in movement', where we change the nature of our support. For instance, when we move from an all fours position to Plank, the moment when the second knee comes off the floor is the moment we can no longer rely on our thigh bone for support, and our muscles instead take up the strain. It is at the *moment of change* that we need to pay most attention, because this is the time when we can find ourselves inadvertently using more effort than required, thereby bringing in unwanted tension. In the end, we need to be able to distinguish between the feeling of our body when it is relaxed, the feeling when we use effort (the *appropriate* amount of work we need to use to

FIND YOUR FEET

There is one thing I practise in almost every class, and that is work on the feet.

There are two main aims here. One is to strengthen and mobilise the feet. This involves squatting on your haunches (up on your toes), resting the arms on the knees, and gently swaying from side to side for a minute or two.

Then there is the matter of 'mapping' the toes. In cultures where it is the norm to wear shoes for much of the day, the toes lose their sensory intelligence. We can help to re-map them by standing and spreading the toes wide, and then lifting all the toes up and then putting them down. Then lifting all the little toes but not the big toe. Then lifting the big toe but not the little ones. If you can do that, move on to try lifting the middle three toes, leaving the little and big toes on the ground. Finally, try moving the big toes towards and away from their neighbouring toes.

In many of the asana descriptions in this book, I talk about 'finding your footprint'. By this I mean the print that is made if the weight is equal on the inner and outer foot, and on the front and back of the foot. People vary in terms of how much of an arch they have, but this is almost immaterial. What is interesting is the way weight falls through the footprint.

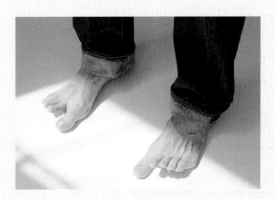

do something) and the feeling when we are holding tension (when we use *more* effort than is required for any given task).

In this sense, there is a difference between those asanas that see us moving from one position to another, or simply moving in and out of them, and those where we are mainly at rest, such as with Child's pose. In the former we get a constant flow of information about how we are feeling and moving; we are provided with sensations to notice. So these types of asanas are especially helpful in our pursuit of 'mapping' ourselves on multiple levels. When we are still and resting, on the other hand, we can concentrate on losing tension by finding support through our bones and the floor. Both types of asana are useful, but for different reasons.

BELOW
Moving asanas, such as Sprinter,
provide a constant flow of information.

NOTICING LEVELS OF DISCOMFORT

Finally, and perhaps most profoundly, we need to be able to notice when we feel in discomfort, and then to respond to that feeling appropriately, if possible. Of course, this is most obvious with any pain that presents itself in our body. If we sit in one position for too long, our body will start to signal its discomfort and it is then sensible to make an adjustment to our position. It may seem odd that many people are not very good at noticing how they feel in their body, but it is often the case that our daily lives lead us away from our bodies and into our heads. Then slowly, over time, we become less good at distinguishing what and how wc feel.

In yoga, we are sometimes encouraged to stretch our muscles to the limit. This is uncomfortable for a reason, and can lead to damage to the muscle/tendon if done too regularly. Movement is good but regularly taking a movement to the end of its range will often result in damage that can take some time to heal.

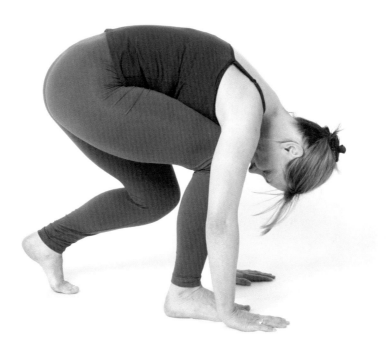

It is worth pointing out that uncomfortable feelings in the body are not always related to our tissues, however. As I explored earlier, uncomfortable emotional feelings are also often felt in the body as we respond to encounters in the outside world, whether it be a knot in the stomach, or tightness in the throat. These, too, are promptings to change our behaviour, requiring us to apologise for a harsh word we let slip in a moment of anger, for instance, or to give vent to feelings of grief and loss that we have found difficult to acknowledge.

SELF-PRACTICE: GETTING ON OUR MATS

There are many reasons why we might decide to get on our yoga mat to practise. We may simply feel a little stiff after a period of inactivity and want to move a bit. Or we might be feeling agitated about something that is going on in our life and feel the need to calm ourselves down. But perhaps the most significant thing about finding some regular time to get on your mat is that it allows your mind to become quiet as you drop into the sensations of the body.

There is no rule as to how much time one should practise. Five minutes may suffice on one day, an hour on another. The important thing is to find a way to incorporate it into your life in some way. (While I type these words, I have a mat by my chair and periodically move to it either for a change of position or to refresh my mind when the words feel stuck.) Over time, a regular practice provides the possibility of more clarity about the things that are getting in the way of fulfilling your potential, in all manner of ways.

If you have room in your living space, keep a mat on the floor and visit it periodically. Start by paying attention to what your felt sense (see p.101 **Introducing a 'felt sense'**) is informing you of. You can lie on your back, or on your side or front. Or you may be in Child's pose. Wait quietly until you want to move, then change position and see how that feels. Then start to notice all the small elements of movement you went through to change position until you have noticed all you can about both the

position and the movement from one position to another. Then you can try again to see how simple and comfortable you can make every aspect of the position and the transition. When noticing changes in sensation becomes something familiar, you might start noticing more clearly the point at which you start to feel anxious when approaching head balance, for instance. Not just noticing that you fear the posture, but becoming clear about *why* you fear the posture. It might be that feeling of weight on your head is uncomfortable. Or you might remember an article you read saying it was dangerous. Once the fear has been identified, you can set about resolving it, but simply being afraid of head balance in some vague way is not helpful at all.

The stripping away of unnecessary noise from your nervous system when you practise yoga allows other noises to become more apparent. Thoughts or feelings of restlessness appear and reappear until we are able to make sense of them. You may have been feeling miserable or unhappy, and slowly come to realise that it is your job or relationship that is the cause, or a particular behaviour that you find difficult to address.

'The stripping away of unnecessary noise from your nervous system when you practise yoga allows other noises to become more apparent.'

———

Once these thoughts or feelings have surfaced, you then have the choice to do something about them. If an uneasy feeling of disquiet goes unacknowledged, it will have continual power over you, rather than you over it. Thus, this approach goes beyond the mat, allowing yoga to permeate our lives.

As calmness is the goal, it is sensible to start your practice with something that quietens you down. When the nervous system is calm, we are able to discern changes in our state more easily, so lying in semi-supine (on your back with both knees bent) or in Child's pose can be a good starting point. If we start from this, there is no need to 'warm up'. Whatever it is we decide to do from that point on, we want to carry as much of the quiet state with us as is possible. When we are clear that we are as quiet as possible, we are noticing ourselves in the moment and we want to stay that way throughout our practice. What we are trying to notice is anything that drags us away from that. It could be the attempt to complete a posture, for instance – this takes us into the future. Or we may anticipate a difficulty in a movement based on an experience we have had in the past. Neither being mentally in the future nor being in the past is helpful to us when we practise. Instead, if we simply notice how we are feeling in any given moment, we are more likely to respond appropriately rather than predictably.

If we are attending to *noticing* rather than to *structure*, there is no real need to hold postures for any length of time – unless, of course, one can quieten into it as with Child's pose. It is more useful to visit the movement and then leave it, or perhaps to repeat it a few times with the intention of seeing whether it can be made simpler, done with less effort. This is significant: the attentive repetition of a movement is how we learn. It is how we map the neural connections for the movement. This cannot happen if we simply stay still in a pose. But if we regularly repeat the movement, this skill can then be taken into everything we do in life.

GROUNDING

The notion of grounding is well known in yoga and other bodywork circles. However, its nature can be somewhat elusive; after all, how can one be more or less on the ground? Clearly we cannot become physically heavier or lighter on command, but we can *feel* that we are. Grounding is a subjective experience of feeling more supported by the floor, which gives us a sense of stability and potential for movement.

Physically, things do happen as a result of our capacity to give the weight of our body to the floor without unnecessary interference from muscles.

Bones are the only structures in the body that receive and transmit linear forces. When we 'find' our bones and allow them to assume a supporting role, muscles can start to relax. It is in the 'undoing' of muscles that freedom in the joints is found – and with it, greater ease in movement.

All posture work should be preceded by a sense of grounding so that we do not carry tension (or 'unnecessary effort') and previously held patterns into our practice. This is a slow but fruitful process, a constant investigation of ways to maintain the integrity of a movement without accumulating tension. It is in this spirit that one should approach all asana work.

CHOOSING WHICH ASANAS

There are no real rules about which postures to practise, but it may be wise over time to make sure that you regularly cover all the movement bases outlined in the asana section of this book, i.e. some extension movements, some flexion movements, some side-bending movements, some rotation movements. It is also a good idea to practise some balances, as well as getting up and down from the floor, and being on the floor in varied forms of sitting. In my own practice I have noticed I might emphasise a theme for several months – exploring extension movements, for example – before shifting to something else. Earlier in my yoga life I think these shifts would have been more rapid. The point really is that you find out something about yourself through these explorations.

Yoga practice should not be seen so much as a discipline as a pleasure. Take your time and do not worry if you only do one or two asanas. The most important thing is to do each asana with your full attention on what you are doing, and to stop as soon as paying attention becomes difficult. You may be surprised at how things develop if you allow yourself to be drawn into your yoga rather than 'practising a routine'.

Over time, if you practise a broad gamut of asanas or movements and pay attention to them while you practise, you start to map your body in richer detail. You become clearer about the sensations you feel and

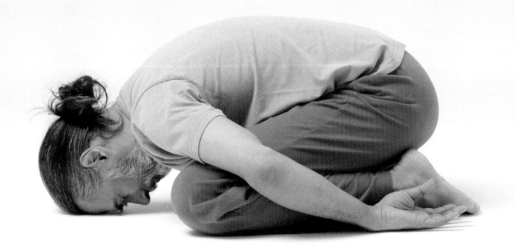

INTRODUCING A 'FELT SENSE'

Whether settling into our practice at home or arriving at a class, it is helpful to try to get into the right frame of mind. In a class, this might involve greeting people and, in the process, gently putting your thoughts in order and adjusting to your surroundings. If practising at home, try to deal with any pressing issues before you start. In both cases it is important to mentally give yourself permission to spend the next moments concentrating on your practice.

It is generally helpful to start a practice with quiet movements and postures. For instance, lying on your back with your knees bent and feet on the floor. This gives you a chance to settle, to arrive in the moment and to pay gentle attention to how the feet are placed on the floor and to the support you feel from the floor through your bones. Or you may want to fold into Child's pose, allowing the joints of the hips, knees and ankles to settle into their end range of movement.

It is not easy to describe the type of attention required to practise yoga, yet it is specific. Imagine you were learning to throw a ball through a basketball hoop. It would be no good just to keep throwing the ball at the hoop in a thoughtless way, with the hopeful expectation that things would improve. To improve your throwing, you would need to gather yourself both mentally and physically. There would be a sense of and focus on what you are doing that is not 'cognitive', but more a 'felt' sense.

In our yoga practice it is this quality of experience that we are trying to generate – an improved quality of feeling that may express itself in a smoother movement or a greater feeling of ease. It may disturb our breathing less and we may feel more stable and more comfortable in ourselves. These things give us clues as to whether the quality of our movement is improving and help us to develop our ability to pay attention to ourselves in the moment.

It is worth adding that when you first start to follow the instructions in the asana descriptions of this book, you may find it hard to fully inhabit your body in this way. The movements may feel a little clunky as you follow the text suggestions. However, once the actions of the particular asana are fully understand, we can then dwell on the felt sense, which develops over time as we become more familiar with what we are doing.

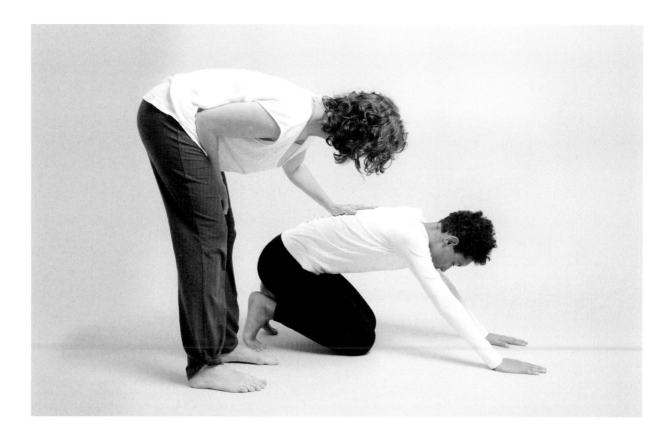

ABOVE
Yoga teachers can try to help students to notice themselves in many different ways.

what your feelings represent. You start to get to know yourself in a sensory way, and as all information about the world arrives through our senses and shapes our nervous system, this is no bad thing.

When we initially meet this approach we may be bemused by its subtleties. This is especially true if we are expecting to do 'exercise', and to some extent it is better to compare this way of working to meditation rather than exercise, because it stops us worrying about how to make it more exciting or interesting. It would be an odd thought to try to make meditation 'exciting', as it is an introspective practice, and as such the mindset needs to be adjusted in that direction. Our allies become curiosity, patience and persistence.

YOGA TEACHING AND CLASSES

Teaching is, of course, different from self-practice. We are working with other people's nervous systems, and we often have little or no idea what has formed

that person. We can be sure that, whatever condition they arrive in when they come into the class, they will have done their best to cope with whatever life has thrown at them. Tensions and holding patterns often develop because of an individual's response to difficult circumstances. We do not tighten our muscles because we feel secure, but quite the opposite. It is important to bear this in mind before we rush to change what we perceive of as 'bad posture'. When we consider this, and fully recognise that a person's posture is simply a representation of their history, it makes less sense to try to 'correct' them. If they have any possibility of change, and indeed if they actually want to change, it is not helpful to suggest that what they are doing is wrong.

What might be helpful, however, is to clarify to them exactly what they are doing and open up some *choices*. For example, if someone is standing in a stooped posture, it might be useful to get him or her to stoop *more*. Their posture is a habituated somatic response, and can no longer be *felt* as a stoop. However, if you exaggerate it, it will be felt again. Then you can go through the whole pattern of stooping (flexion) and reverse your way out of it towards extension. If you do this several times, you start to recognise that you are held in one 'frame' of a movement pattern.

We can play with similar movements lying down, sitting, standing and on all fours, until the person slowly recognises that choices are available. Over months and years, sensory feedback will tend to lead people back to something more efficient and useful. This will not be a 'correction' to their faulty posture, however. It will be a genuine response to how they are feeling in the moment. The point is not so much to try to give someone good posture, more to allow them to have the posture they need for the circumstances they are in.

When we, as yoga teachers, run regular classes, what we teach may depend on the type of class we hold. A drop-in class will be different from a class where people come for a term. In the latter, the teacher might want to work through a theme for a few weeks until they feel that the students have a grasp of what they are talking about. For instance, helping people notice the relationship between breathing and movement is something that is quite subtle, and might not become clear in just one lesson. With a drop-in class, it might be more sensible to cover a wider range of movements and asanas so that students get a better overall sense of what you are teaching.

There is another aspect to teaching a class that can feel a bit tricky, and it is to do with the mereological fallacy referred to in the introduction and chapter one. We know that, in life, when we think about doing something, we do not generally separate the task down to parts of the body. For instance, if I want to put my shoe on in the morning, I simply bend down to reach my foot and put the shoe on. I do not think about engaging this or that muscle, or moving one bit of my body instead of another bit. Tasks or intentions talk to the body as a whole, not to individual parts, and we should reflect this in our yoga classes. So, if students are on all fours and the teacher gives the instruction to 'look up', what we want to find out is whether a person's whole body understands this instruction, or whether only the neck responds. If we tell the body *how* to look up by instructing it – saying, for instance, 'Send the tail

bone to the ceiling and dip your back down' – all you really find out is how good people are at following instructions… which is not very helpful. If, however, we notice that when we give the instruction to look up, a student's pelvis does not move, then there are a few things we can consider. Firstly, it might be that the student thought you meant that they were only allowed to move the neck. Yoga has become very prescriptive, and many styles 'micro-manage' the body. If we are teaching people who are used to that way of working, we might need to be explicit about saying that they can move whatever or however they need to. If it seems that they have understood that, and the pelvis still does not move when the student is asked to look up, we can suspect that they are 'holding' it in some way. It would then be worth the teacher giving a different instruction to encourage the pelvis to participate – for example 'Imagine you have a tail and are wagging it up and down.' Once the student 'finds' their pelvis, it is more likely to join in. The aim is to help them integrate the head and pelvis into the movement rather than simply getting them to follow instructions. When we respond spontaneously and efficiently with the whole body to an instruction to move, it is considered to be a 'compliant' response. The more compliant our body is in life, the better.

Remember, we are not teaching 'exercise', we are trying to help people notice themselves in many different ways. So it is more useful to pose interesting questions about their responses to an invitation to move, rather than to give them a list of instructions to follow.

As I explained above, I am a believer in repetition as a means to refine and improve a movement, and a question that often comes up in relation to this is, 'Don't people get bored with doing the same thing over and over again?' I don't think they do, particularly, if you frame the idea of practice well. If you approach yoga with an 'exercise' attitude, boredom may well be the outcome. If, however, you view it as more like learning an instrument or new skill, it can become endlessly fascinating, as more of ourselves comes into view.

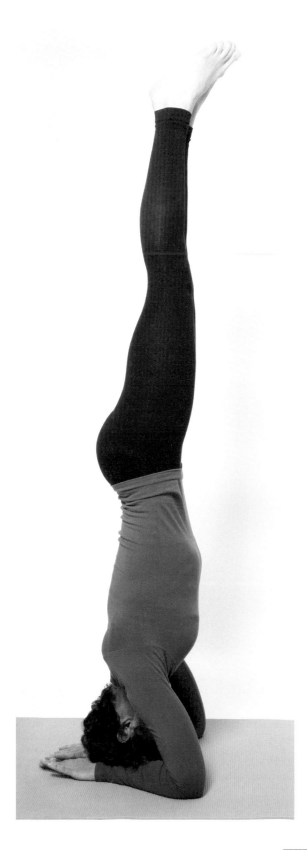

USING THIS BOOK

In the following sections on postures I will be looking at the asanas from a purely human perspective, to the best of my understanding, rather than following any specific tradition. I have divided the asanas up into families of movement. So, **flexion**, **extension**, **side-bending** and **rotation** are all in their own categories, as are **sitting asanas**, **balances** and **tension-losing** asanas. There may be some surprises, as I include Head balance, a classic balance, in tension-noticing poses, as well as Wheel, which would normally be thought of primarily as an extension posture. I have tried to explain my reasons in the text that accompanies each pose.

My intention is to make these asanas as beneficial as possible by explaining the biomechanics involved and, more importantly, our reasons for doing them. As I stated before, unless we have a clear understanding of why we are doing something, it is very difficult to know if we are doing it well or badly. It is important not to try to imitate these postures too literally, but to see them as inadequate representations, or static images, of expansion, contraction and motion – of living patterns of movement.

I have also elected, wherever possible, to use descriptive English titles for postures in preference to more widely used English and Sanskrit names. This is in a bid to avoid ambiguity and to clarify the purpose of the asana.

Lastly, I would also like to make the point that the practice section of this book is not meant to be a collection of rules. Rather, these are principles that can inform one's yoga practice. Rules can lead to dogma, they can dull one's capacity to think. The less we understand, the more hidebound we are by rules. A principle, on the other hand, can deepen one's understanding.

LEFT
Learning how to quieten yourself is an important intention when practising Head Balance.

A CRITIQUE OF SOME MODERN YOGA ASANAS

As I mentioned in the opening chapters of this book, yoga has been with us in the West for more than 50 years. Yoga posture work today comes in many different forms and systems, and it is up to the individual to decide the style that best suits him or her. However, there are a few commonly taught postures that I am outlining here that can cause significant joint problems in those who practise them regularly. The chief culprits are Warrior One, with the back foot turned out, and Triangle posture. I also mention below some other postures that I no longer teach, either because they can be anatomically damaging, or simply because they are fairly pointless from my perspective.

WARRIOR ONE
(Virabhadrasana I)
The first problem to consider with this asana is what happens to the knee of the back leg. If this asana is taught with the foot of the back leg turned out by about 30 degrees, and the hip facing forward, two things will inevitably happen: the arch of the foot will collapse, and a rotational force will be put through the knee. Neither of these things is in any way useful, and what happens to the knee is potentially dangerous. The cartilage in the knee does not enjoy

BELOW
Compression of the lumbar spine in Warrior One.

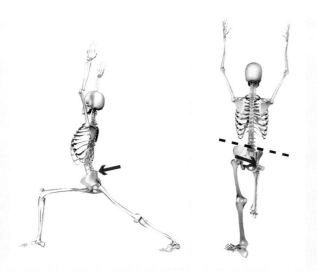

rotational forces. In fact, repeated rotational stress through the knee can eventually tear the cartilage.

Secondly, we need to look at what is happening in the lower back in this asana. When we take a wide forward stride, facing the front leg, the iliopsoas and iliofemoral ligaments are tensioned to their limit. This pulls the pelvis into an anterior tilt, compressing the lumbar spine (see bottom left). The tighter the structures (either ligament or muscle) at the front of the hip, the greater the compression on the back of the spine. If the hip is stiff, the pelvis cannot come forwards enough and this hip will then be higher than the other one. This will introduce side bending and rotation into the lower spine (see bottom right) while it is under compression – a recipe for disaster. A solution is to turn the back foot to face forwards. This takes torsion out of the knee and helps the hip come round slightly. But the stride also needs to be narrowed for most people so that the pelvis and, therefore, the lumbar spine, can be brought into a stress-free alignment. I explain the asana in full on page 136.

Turning the back foot out in any forward-facing asana – such as Stepping-forward Forward Bend (Parsvottanasana), Warrior one and Reverse Triangle (Parivrtta Trikonasana) – presents similar problems for the knees. Most students simply do not have the freedom in their hips to remove strain at the knee. Although I have been taught many variations of these types of postures, nothing solves the problem as well as pointing both hips and feet in the same direction, and, perhaps surprisingly, very little if anything is lost in terms of the stretch offered by the posture.

TRIANGLE
(Trikonasana)
This posture is often taught with the leading foot (right one in illustration) turned to 90 degrees and the back foot to 45 degrees. The teacher might then ask the student to imagine that the entire body is in contact with a wall behind them, so that the movement in the spine is pure side-bending.

However, as the left hip is taken back towards

the 'wall', the right knee will inevitably roll inwards, putting an unnecessary and unhelpful rotational force through the knee (see top image below). To make the side bend safe for the knee it actually makes much more sense to keep both feet, both knees and the spine facing forwards (see middle image below).

Some teachers allow the hip of the 'back' leg – i.e. the leg on the opposite side to the one which you

BELOW
Unhelpful rotational forces in Triangle.

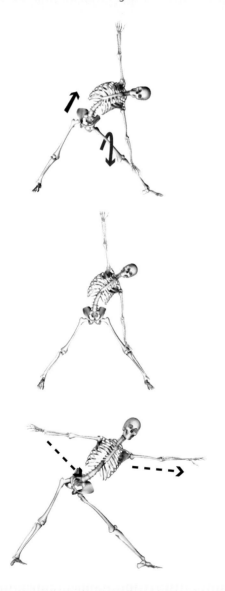

are bending towards – to drift forwards and the hip of the front leg to drop (see bottom image below). This reduces rotation and, therefore, stress on the knee joint, making the posture safe. Now, however, the pose is merely a mild twist in the spine and a gentle stretch in the leg. It becomes pointless.

It is sometimes suggested that the arm should stretch sideways while the hip drops, allowing the underside waist to lengthen. This may be fine for people with very flexible hips, but those with stiffer hips risk injury to the lower back by doing this. When the spine is asked to lengthen sideways, the movement can be accommodated to some extent by the individual joints and discs of the spine. At some point, though, the sideways movement meets the lumbosacral and sacroiliac joints, which are relatively fixed in place, so it imposes a shearing force on them. If this asana is to have any meaning then you have to first clarify what it is you are teaching. Is it a side bend or a twist? In a sense it does not matter which it is, as long as you are clear about what you are doing. I tend to approach this as a twist, as I describe on page 161.

V-SITTING
(Paripuna navasana)
Though the first edition of this book included V-sitting, or full Boat pose, it no longer fits into the way I am thinking about yoga. It is mainly about strengthening the hip flexors, but in a way that is never used in normal life, i.e. to help us hold our legs up in front of us.

One of the more interesting things about the group of muscles that make up the hip flexors is its role in maintaining and modifying the lumbar curve as we move about in daily life. So it is much more useful to map the way this group of muscles modifies the lumbar curve as described in the supine tension-losing asanas on pages 112 and 113.

I feel similarly about the Half Boat posture that I included in the first edition. Simply trying to strengthen the abdominal wall by holding a modified sit-up is again reductionist and unhelpful. It is always better to clarify function than to target a muscle.

STRAIGHT-LEGGED SITTING

Omitting straight-legged sitting asanas like Staff pose (Dandasana) and Wide-legged sitting (Upavistha Konasana) is probably a bit more contentious. But these are particularly miserable postures for anyone with tight hamstrings, and very few people will choose this way of sitting in daily life unless they have long hamstrings. I do realise that these asanas can be modified, but I see little point in helping someone to practise a movement that they are very unlikely to choose in life when more helpful alternatives are available.

For many years, the yoga world has for some reason pursued the notion that having long hamstrings is automatically beneficial, seeming to forget that bending a knee resolves most limitations imposed by tight hamstrings. Sitting movements and postures that ask the hips to rotate and the knees to bend, as any crossed-legged postures do – including Gomukhasana, or the Yin-style Deer pose – are more beneficial to the hips, knees, feet and ankles, as they are being asked to participate in the movement, which is not the case in straight-legged sitting asanas.

I am happy to make a compromise with the one-legged variations of straight-legged sitting, however, because here we can emphasise what is going on with the other hip. We can, for example, straighten the left leg away and fold the right leg into various sitting positions, such as Half Cobbler

BELOW
There are often better alternatives to straight-legged sitting.

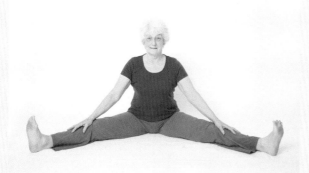

pose (Janusirsasana), Half Hero (Triang Mukha Eka Pada Paschimottanasana) and Half Lotus (Eka Pada Baddha Paschimottanasana). However, if the hamstrings of the long leg are a little tight, it is important to do these postures with your back against a wall. This is because if we try to maintain a reasonably straight spine when we have tight hamstrings, we will inevitably engage the iliopsoas muscle to 'hold our spine up'. And because this muscle also flexes the hip, it is impossible to release the hip joint fully when it is trying to hold us upright. If we put our back to the wall, however, the iliopsoas can relax, so the hip joint can also relax and the folded leg has more freedom to move.

OTHER ASANAS I NO LONGER TEACH

There are several other asanas that are often taught in modern yoga classes that I no longer teach. These include the more intense, straight-legged version of **Standing Forward Bend** (*Uttanasana*); **Chair pose** (*Utkatasana*); and **Warrior Two** (*Virabhadrasana II*).

When Uttanasana is taught with straight legs, with the intention of stretching the hamstrings, it serves no useful purpose. And as I have mentioned before, stretching for the sake of it gets you nowhere. However, taken as a flexion movement, where the spine and knees participate, this asana becomes more useful, as I have explained on page 146.

Chair pose, on the other hand, is almost always a stress position. It almost always tightens people up in the muscles that are usually too tight anyway, particularly the lower erector spinae and the iliopsoas. I therefore do not teach this asana at all.

Although Warrior Two is a very popular pose for many yoga practitioners, and not much can go wrong anatomically, it is also a little pointless. There is no meaningful movement of the spine, and the actions of the legs and hips are really just about stretching the adductors. As discussed before, stretching a muscle does not change the way it functions in the body, because the action does not relate to anything done in normal life by the vast majority of people.

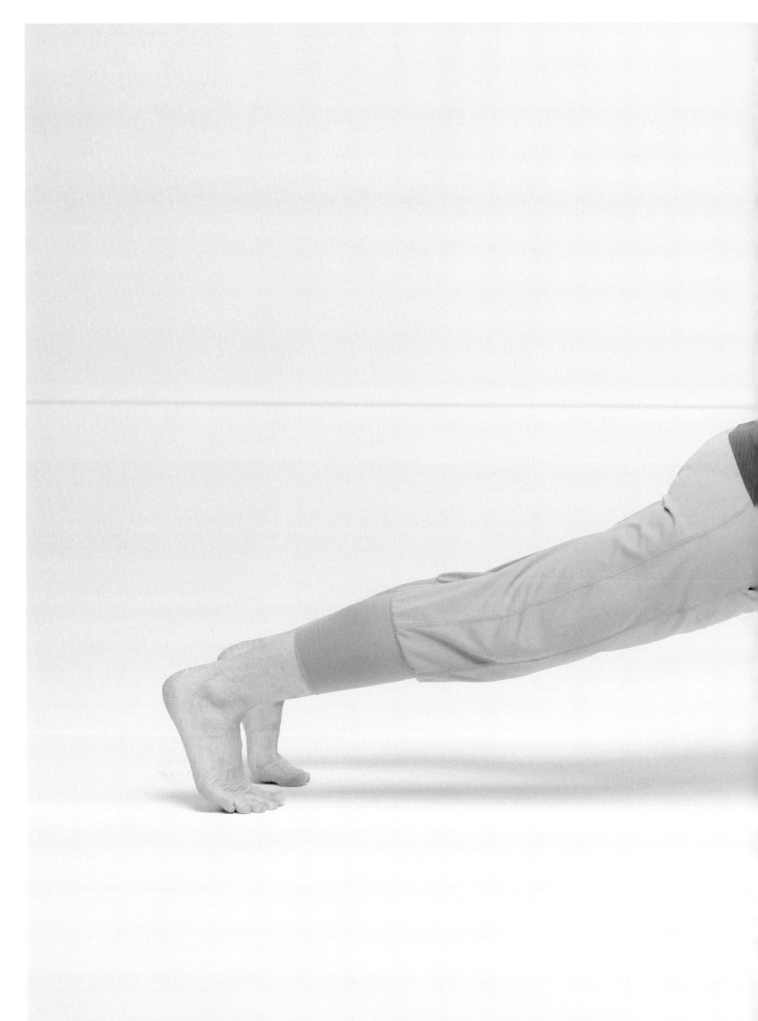

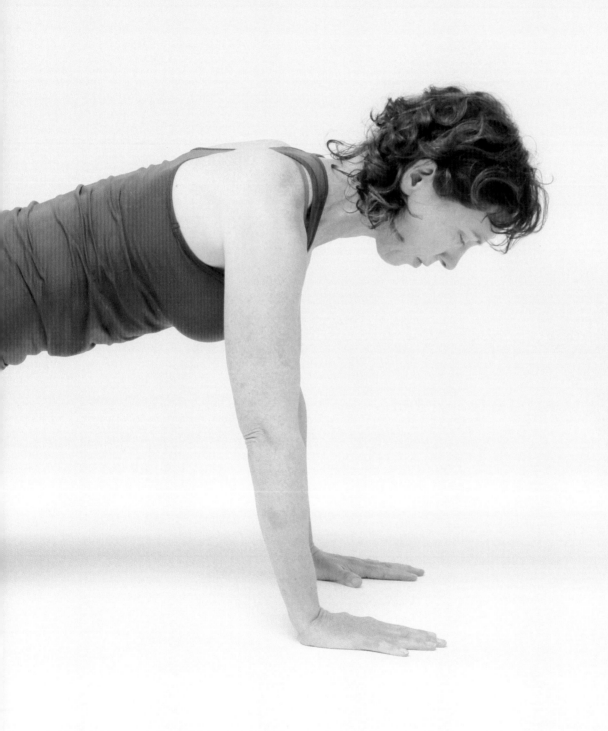

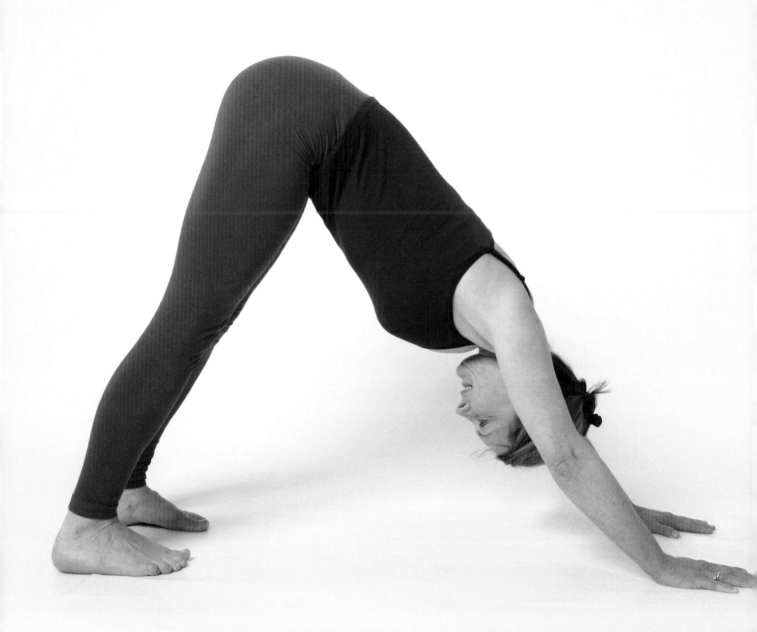

SEVEN

TENSION-LOSING ASANAS

Although I approach most yoga posture and movement work around the idea of functional movement, some asanas are clearly not 'functional' in terms of daily life. Headstand, Dog pose and Plank, for example, have very little to do with everyday function. So, why practise them?

I would argue that these postures just mentioned, and others included in this section, have another, distinct purpose. They offer an opportunity for us to learn to differentiate the feeling of a relaxed muscle from that of a working muscle, and also that of a working muscle from a tense muscle.

This group of postures has a precise purpose: to help us find support for the body through the skeleton and the floor to reduce muscular effort. Using bones, as opposed to muscles, requires no 'effort'; and when we arrange our bones skillfully, muscles then have less work to do. It is not that muscles then have *no* work to do, but they will have less work. And in terms of efficiency, that is advantageous.

What we learn when we practise like this is how to reduce habitually held tension. Habitual tension is very difficult to spot because, as it is so familiar, it feels like 'us'. It feels normal. So we have to learn what support feels like, what effort feels like, and what tension feels like. It is rarely a question of, 'Am I doing the posture "right"?' What is more useful to ask is, 'Do I know how it feels?'

IN THIS SECTION

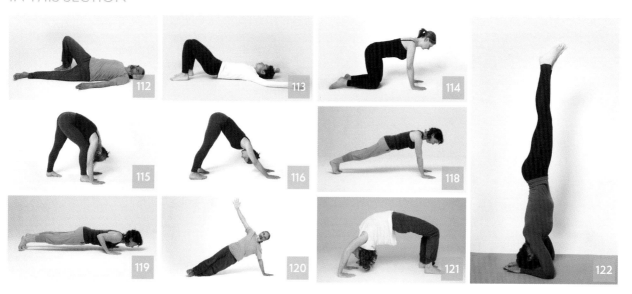

PRESSING ONE FOOT INTO THE FLOOR

A note on the footprint: this is the print that would be made if the weight were equal on the inner and outer foot, and on the front and the back of the foot. People vary in terms of how much of an arch they have, but this is almost immaterial. What I am concerned with is the way weight falls through the footprint.

PURPOSE

- To 'map' the effective organisation of the active leg pushing down into the floor, and to map the contact area of the footprint on the floor.
- To notice any stiffening in the trunk and resting leg as the active leg pushes into the floor. To also notice any changes to our breathing as the active leg pushes into the floor.

APPROACHING THE ASANA

1. Start by lying on your back (supine) on the floor, with legs straight, and relaxing. Bend your right knee and bring the sole of your foot to the floor. Spend a little time finding the very best place for the foot so that it can press into the floor with maximum efficiency. Be sure that the whole footprint is represented on the floor and stays that way throughout the movement. Keep the arms relaxed on the floor by your side.
2. Keep your body completely relaxed as you start to press your right foot into the floor, keeping the footprint steady and even throughout. Notice how the consequences of your efforts travel through the body. How, as the foot presses down, your right hip gradually lifts off the floor whilst the left hip stays relaxed on the floor.
3. Gently lower your right hip back down to the floor. Pay attention to the smoothness and flow of the movement. Ensure the right footprint stays well represented throughout the movement.
4. Repeat the movement slowly and smoothly several times, always attempting to become softer in the body. Then repeat on the other side.

SENSE OF ENQUIRY

- Can you feel the whole of the footprint on the ground throughout the movement? Or has the weight shifted to the inner foot?
- Does your breathing stay easy and light throughout the movement?
- Does the raising and lowering of the hip feel smooth and fluid? If not, is there a way you can make it more so?
- Does the relaxed leg remain heavy and resting on the floor? Does the foot of the resting leg move?

Remember, the only instruction is to press your foot into the floor as described. Everything that happens as a result is simply a *consequence*, not an *intention*.

PRESSING BOTH FEET INTO THE FLOOR
(BRIDGE)

Setu Bandha Sarvangasana

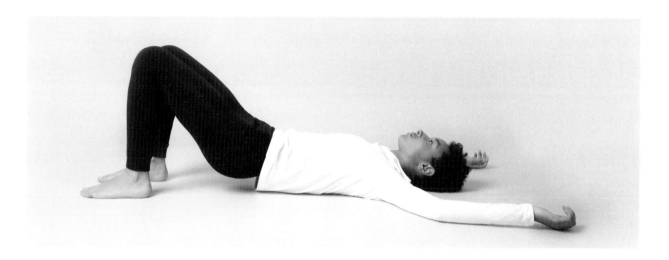

PURPOSE

- To map the effective organisation of the legs pushing into the floor, and the contact of the feet to the floor as you push down.
- To try to notice any stiffening of the trunk as you push the feet into the floor. This is best noticed by the way the pelvis and spine leave the floor. If the body is really relaxed, the pelvis will come off the floor first followed by the spine, which may feel like it is coming off vertebra by vertebra. If there is tension in the trunk you will notice the spine and pelvis come off the floor more in a 'block'.

APPROACHING THE ASANA

1. Start by lying on the floor and relaxing. Bring the arms to the floor behind your head, if this is comfortable. Take them wider, if necessary, to find comfort. Bend both knees, bringing both feet to the floor. Find the best place for the feet to press effectively down into the floor. Do not simply be satisfied with your first attempt.
2. When you have found the most useful place, start to press both feet into the floor through the whole footprints, whilst doing your best to remain completely relaxed in your trunk. Observe the very first consequence of pressing into your feet, and follow the consequences through your body.

3. See if you can pause at these staging points: a. When your lower back settles into the floor, i.e. the lumbar curve starts to flatten. b. When the sacrum and back of the pelvis are lifted off the floor but the lumbar spine is still on the floor. c. When the lumbar spine is fully off the floor but the thoracic spine is still on the floor.
4. Lower the pelvis gently back down to the floor and rest before repeating slowly and smoothly several times. Remember that the movement of the pelvis is the *consequence* of pressing your feet into the floor. It is not an intention.

SENSE OF ENQUIRY

- Make sure you are pressing down into your whole footprint rather than pushing your feet away or pressing into only part of the footprint.
- Does your breathing stay easy and light throughout the movement? Or does it change in some way? It might help to observe whether your tummy tightens when you start to press your feet down, or whether you start to hold your breath.
- Does your body stay soft and relaxed throughout the movement? Pay particular attention to the abdomen. If it is relaxed there will be a slight sense that the abdominal wall sinks a little as the movement develops.

FINDING SUPPORT ON ALL FOURS

When we are on all fours, we are supported by four vertical columns. The pelvis is supported by the femurs (thigh bones), so the muscles of the legs have very little work to do if they are organised well. Support through the arms, however, is more complex because there are three areas of variability: the elbows, wrists and the shoulder girdle. So we have to pay more attention to the way we place our hands and arms to get the most efficient support.

When we come onto all fours, we unconsciously choose how we organise the relationship between the scapular and the rib cage. Some people tend to sink a little in this area, others to 'push through' a little. This is simply to do with the way they have mapped the relationship between the scapula and rib cage. There is no 'right' and 'wrong' position, so there is nothing to 'correct'. However, if you are a long way in either direction, it is possible that it will impact on whatever else you do from this position, so it can be useful to explore all the possible relationships that exist here.

For some people, wrists are an issue – they may be stiff or arthritic. In such cases a lift under the heel of the hand can be helpful. It is also useful to change the position of the hands regularly if they are uncomfortable, rather than stay in the same position with pain.

PURPOSE
- To find the most appropriate support, through the legs, lumbar spine, arms and shoulder girdle.
- To map out the choices of support between the scapula and the rib cage.

APPROACHING THE ASANA
1. Come onto all fours and start by simply noticing the support through your arms and legs.
2. Have your elbows fairly straight but not locked, and your hands roughly below the shoulders. If we bend our elbows too much we lose the bones as a means of support, as forces travel in straight lines.
3. Then, slowly sink as far as you can between your shoulders. Then go the other way and push into the floor until your chest is as far from the floor as possible. Go smoothly from one extreme to the other, noticing how it feels as you move.
4. Focus on your pelvis. Tuck it under as if you were putting your tail between your legs. Then go in the other direction so that your lower back hollows. Move smoothly and slowly between these positions.
5. Finally, settle on something that feels useful to you. Try not to intellectualise it by trying to get it 'right' by having a straight spine. Much better to settle on what *feels* okay after some exploration.

SENSE OF ENQUIRY
- Do you feel comfortable across the shoulders?
- Do your hands meet the floor effectively with the weight well distributed?
- How does your neck feel?

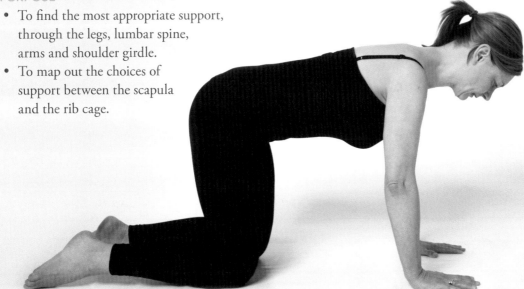

SPRINTER

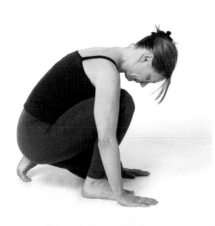 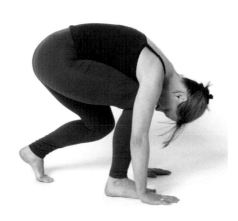 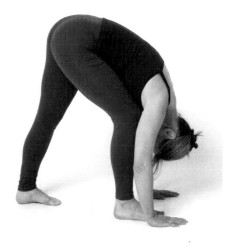

PURPOSE

- To help maintain the strength required in the legs to lift your body weight.
- To put the foot, ankle, knee and hip through the range of movement needed when getting to the floor and back up again.
- To map the movement of the legs whilst the foot is well represented on the floor.
- To help us notice when we bring unnecessary work into the trunk.

PURPOSE

- To help maintain the strength required in the legs to lift your body weight.
- To put the foot, ankle, knee and hip through the range of movement needed when getting to the floor and back up again.
- To map the movement of the legs whilst the foot is well represented on the floor.
- To help us notice when we bring unnecessary work into the trunk.

APPROACHING THE ASANA

1. Come on to all fours and find the appropriate support through your shoulders (see p.114).
2. Tuck your toes under. Bring the right foot forward so that the heel of the right foot is roughly in line with your left knee. Map the whole footprint on the floor.
3. Rest the weight of your pelvis through your right foot and rest your trunk on your right thigh. Rest your hands on the floor on either side of you (more for stability than to take weight).

4. Pause for a moment to check you are as relaxed as possible in this position, then slowly straighten your back leg until the sole of the foot is on the floor, if possible. Keep your trunk resting on your right thigh throughout.
5. Slowly bend your leg again until you are back to your starting position. Repeat several times and then on the other side.

SENSE OF ENQUIRY

- Can you keep your foot well mapped on the floor throughout the movement?
- Can you keep your trunk and neck relaxed throughout the movement?
- Are the movements you make smooth and fluid?
- Is your breathing easy and free throughout the movement?
- Can you make a well-balanced footprint with the back foot when the leg straightens?
- Keep noticing if you are starting to lift your head or tense your neck at any point.

DOWNWARD-FACING DOG

Adho Mukha Svanasana

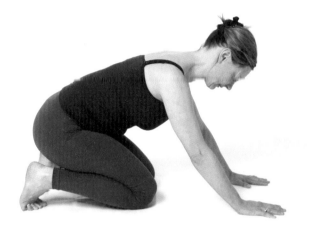 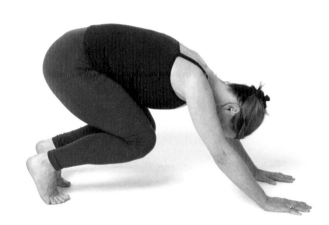

PURPOSE

- To learn to organise effective support through the arms by looking for skeletal support and muscular release across the shoulders.
- To learn to use the legs rather than the arms to lift the pelvis.
- To help free up the respiratory system.
- To help develop the strength in the legs to lift your body weight.

'Do your hands keep a "knowing" contact to the floor throughout the movement?'

APPROACHING THE ASANA

1. Start on all fours, and find your appropriate support through the shoulders (see p.114). Make space between the fingers and distribute the weight evenly across the base of the fingers, if possible.

2. Tuck your toes under and take your weight back onto your heels. At this point, find a way to rest: let your pelvis rest on your heels; let your body feel supported through the arms. Try to find a sense of *leaning* into your hands but not collapsing or pushing.

3. Lift your knees about an inch off the floor. Notice the change in effort. Are you still leaning into your hands or did you start pushing? Can you tell the difference? Find out what the minimum effort is to lift your knees an inch off the floor. The effort of bringing the knees off

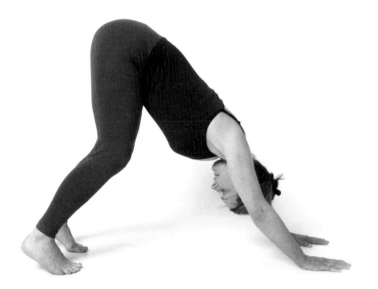
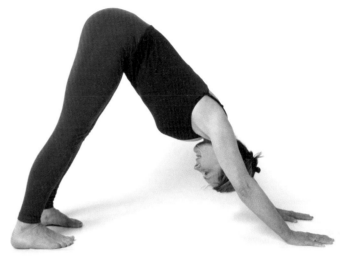

the floor will be distributed throughout the body. The aim is to find the minimum effort required.

4. Once you have done that, slowly start to straighten your legs. As you do so, notice whether you start pushing with your arms, as opposed to feeling supported by them.

5. If your hamstrings are tight, do not straighten your legs completely or you will find yourself having to push back with your arms, causing you to work harder with your shoulders than is helpful. Keep the knees bent enough to allow a reasonably relaxed shoulder girdle with a rough straight line between hands, shoulders and hips. When these points line up you get maximum skeletal support.

SENSE OF ENQUIRY

- Do your hands keep a 'knowing' contact to the floor throughout the movement?
- Can you keep your neck relaxed even when the knees come off the floor?
- Breathing will change a little when the knees come off the floor. Try not to hold or strain your breath at this point.
- A relaxed line from hands through the shoulders to the pelvis is more important than having straight legs.
- If your heels reach the floor, can they make a good footprint?
- Remember that what we are concerned with in Dog is finding useful support through the arms whilst lifting the pelvis with the legs. The arms support the trunk and the legs do the lifting.

PLANK POSE
Kumbhakasana

PURPOSE

- To help check you have sufficient strength in the arms and trunk to support your body weight.
- To bring your attention to the relationship between skeletal support and muscular effort.
- To help map the position of the pelvis in space when the legs stop supporting it.

APPROACHING THE ASANA

1. Start by coming onto all fours. Then take your hands a good hand's length further forward. Find the appropriate support through your shoulders. Notice the position of your pelvis in space.
2. Very carefully straighten out your right leg, being watchful to keep the pelvis from moving too much.
3. When you start to straighten the left leg, you will notice the body's uptake of muscular effort at the point at which the left knee leaves the floor. Keep your effort to a minimum whilst maintaining the position of the pelvis in space. Notice the feeling of change in the body's state once both knees have left the floor. Stay for a short moment and then bring the knees back to the floor. Notice again how the feeling of the body changes.
4. Repeat slowly two or more times. Each time, see how surreptitiously you can take the knees off the floor. Imagine you could take the knees off the floor without the shoulders finding out!

SENSE OF ENQUIRY

- Does the position of the pelvis change when you take your knees off the floor?
- What is the least effort you need to maintain to keep the pelvis in place when the knees come off the floor?
- In what way does your breathing change when your knees come off the floor?

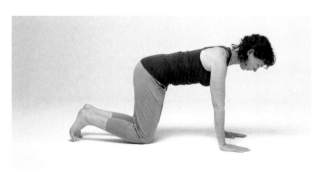 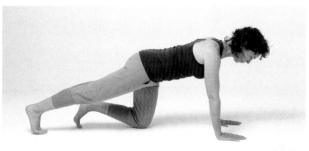

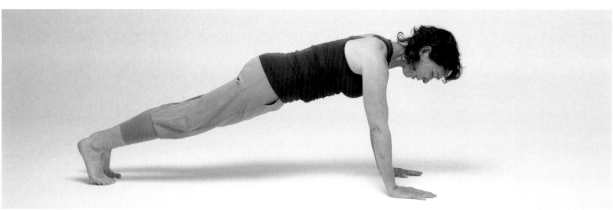

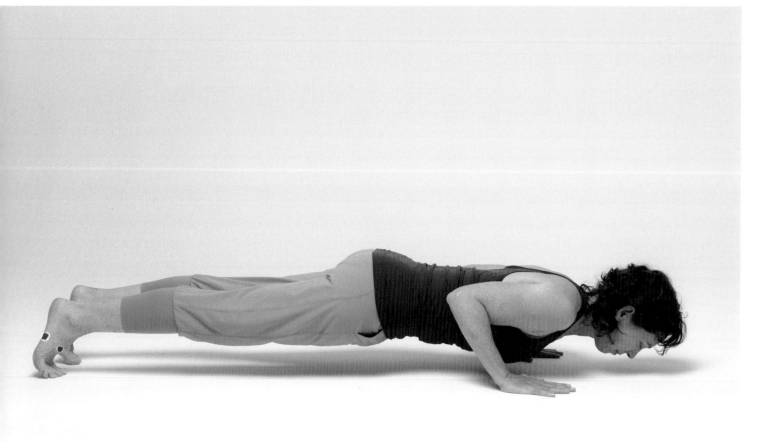

BENT-ARM PLANK

Chaturanga Dandasana

PURPOSE
- To help check whether you have the strength in your arms and shoulders to support your body weight.
- To bring your attention to the relationship between skeletal support and muscular effort.
- To help map the position of the body as muscular effort increases.

APPROACHING THE ASANA
1. Come into Plank as described on p.118. Notice the straightness of your body.
2. Start to bend the elbows whilst keeping a reasonable handprint on the floor. As you bend your elbows you are no longer able to use the bones in your arms as a means of support, and the muscles of your arms and shoulder girdle have to take up more work, as do all the muscles on the front of the body. Notice the change in the feeling state of your body as your elbows bend. Do your best to maintain the feeling of straightness through your body. Do not stay for any length of time.
3. If you have the energy, you can repeat slowly a few more times, trying to reduce the effort involved each time.

SENSE OF ENQUIRY
- Did you notice whether the body moved away from its straight line or not?
- Could you maintain a good handprint on the floor throughout the movement?
- Did the position of the shoulders change significantly throughout the movement?

SIDE PLANK

Vasisthasana

PURPOSE
- To look for skeletal support in slightly more complex circumstances.
- To map the position of the pelvis.
- To check you have the strength in your trunk to maintain the position of your pelvis. (Note that it is pointless trying to name the muscles involved, as almost every muscle on the front of your trunk will be involved.)

APPROACHING THE ASANA
1. Come into Plank as described on p.118, and notice the position of your pelvis.
2. Turn the feet so the outside of the left foot is on the ground and the inside of the right foot is on the ground.
3. Bring the right hand off the floor and turn the body to face the right wall. Then, lift your right arm. Notice whether the pelvis drops or lifts from the midline.
4. The feet can either simply turn, in which case the right foot will be in front of the left; or, you can bring the right foot to rest on top of the left foot.
5. Try playing around with the position of the upper hand. When the arm lines up with your collarbone, you will find you get the best skeletal support (this tends to be when the arm is at about a right angle to the trunk), which will reduce the muscular activity of the arm and shoulder.

SENSE OF ENQUIRY
- Can you notice that there is a best position for the supporting hand?
- Can you tell whether the pelvis had moved up or down as you turned?
- How did your breathing change as your body turned?

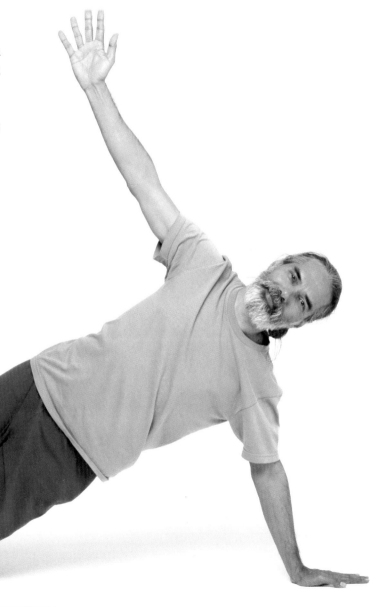

WHEEL

Urdhva Dhanurasana

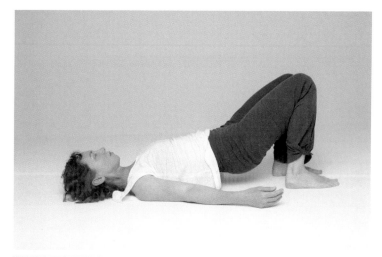

This posture is understandably usually classed as a back bend because the shape is undeniably one of extension. However, there is no *active* back bending going on in this posture at all. In fact, any active back-bending of the spine can be counter-productive, particularly if the lower ribs start to lift too early in the movement. This has the effect of creating anterior rotation of the pelvis, the opposite of what is needed in this movement.

PURPOSE

- To help map the best organisation of the feet and hands to push effectively into the floor.
- To practise keeping the trunk as relaxed as possible, whilst the effort of pushing into the floor increases.

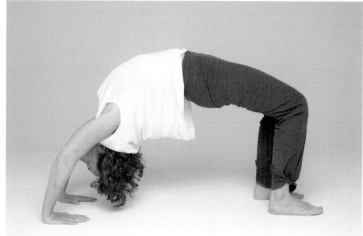

APPROACHING THE ASANA

1. Lie on your back, bend your knees and bring both feet to the floor. Spend a little time to find the best place for your feet to press down into the floor. Map both footprints on the floor until you are sure the feet and legs are in the very best place for pushing down. If it is comfortable, bring your arms over your head and relax them on the floor.

2. Start by gently pressing your feet into the floor until you feel the back of the waist settle into the floor. Gradually continue to press down with your feet until you feel the pelvis lift off the floor. Keep as soft as you can in the body and keep 'standing down' into the legs. Raise your pelvis until it will not go any higher.

3. Bring the hands into the pushing-down position. Find a place where as much of the hands can be on the floor as possible with the elbows pointing towards the ceiling. Press firmly down into your handprints. The transition between resting your head and shoulders on the floor and straightening your arms is the moment that requires the most effort, as you have least skeletal support at that time.

4. Keep breathing as evenly as you can and allow the shoulders to lift until your arms are fairly straight. If you find you cannot lift off without stiffening and holding the breath, simply lower yourself down again. Remember you are practising noticing how you are feeling, and keeping the feeling as comfortable as possible. You are not 'performing' a posture.

5. When you come down, see if you can 're-wind the film' and come down by simply reversing the way you went up.

SENSE OF ENQUIRY

- Once you have found the best position for the feet, can you keep your footprints well mapped throughout the movement?
- Can you keep your breathing appropriate to the effort required?
- Notice the lower front ribs. Can you keep them relaxed and dropping rather than lifting throughout the movement?
- Can you find the most useful place for the hands and arms to push down into the floor?

HEAD BALANCE

Sirasana

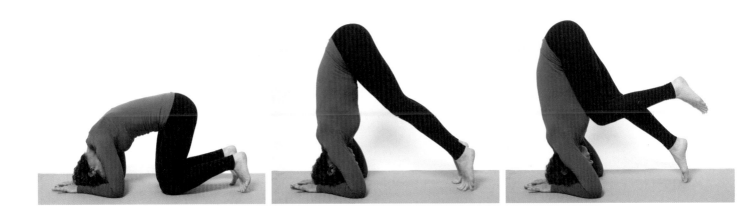

I would like to make it clear that it is not at all important whether you ever manage to get your feet off the floor in this asana. It is a complex posture because its constraints are rarely strength or flexibility. Rather they are to do with your ability to organise yourself well in relation to your contact with the floor.

PURPOSE

- To learn how to quieten yourself through finding useful support through your arms and head, even as the movement becomes more complex.
- To help you notice at what stage you bring unhelpful tension to the movement.
- To help you learn when to stop!

APPROACHING THE ASANA

1. Start by coming into Child's pose (see p.145), with the forehead resting on the floor and your arms beside you. Make sure it is really resting.
2. Lift your bottom off your heels and roll onto the crown of the head. Then roll back onto your heels. Repeat this a few times and make

absolutely sure the head is rolling and not sliding on the floor. Keep your arms beside you.

3. The next time you roll onto the crown of the head, bring the elbows to the floor in a place where you feel you can take some weight through them. Have the wrists close to the head, with the palms of your hands facing more downward than upward. Keep your fingers loose and relaxed.

4. When you have arranged the arms in the best position for support, tuck your toes under and straighten your legs. Notice whether you still feel supported through the arms. If you do not, come down again and try a slightly different place with the elbows. Then try again. If you really cannot maintain good support through the elbows when you straighten the legs, do not go any further. Just practise this stage.

5. If you can maintain good support through the elbows when you straighten your legs, start to walk the feet towards you until they begin to feel light – at which point you can bring the feet off the floor. Do your very best to smooth out the

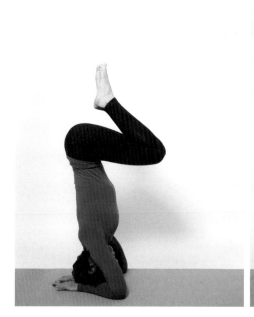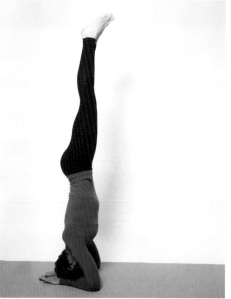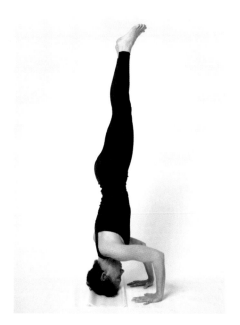

transition between the point when the feet are on the floor and when they come off the floor. Folding at the knees as you bring your feet off the floor usually eases the transition.

THREE-POINT VARIATION (FAR RIGHT)

1. In the three-point variation of Head Balance, you start in a similar way by coming into Child's pose and then rolling onto the crown of the head and back again, until you have familiarised yourself with the feeling.

2. Then bring your hands to the floor roughly on either side of your knees, so that the heel of each hand is approximately in line with the front of your knees. When you roll onto the crown of your head, be sure the hands stay very well grounded – especially the base of the thumbs.

3. Keep your attention on maintaining a good handprint on the floor as you straighten your legs. If you find you cannot do this then do not go any further. Simply practise the movements up to this point. If all is well and you can straighten your legs whilst maintaining a steady handprint, you can bring one knee up onto your forearm – again, this should not feel awkward or a strain. If it does, do not go any further. But if you feel okay then bring the other knee onto the other forearm and again check you feel stable and quiet. Only if you feel quite at home in this position is it worth trying to straighten your legs towards the ceiling. Remember the point is to maintain a sense of quiet equilibrium rather than simply getting your legs straight.

SENSE OF ENQUIRY

- Can you maintain your whole handprint on the floor, particularly the inner hand and base of the thumb as you straighten your legs? If you manage this, your elbows will be in the right place.

- Did your head roll onto the crown as you straightened your legs? Or did it slide a bit? If there was some sliding, it implies that there is some tension in your neck.

- Did you hold or shorten your breath at any point during the movement?

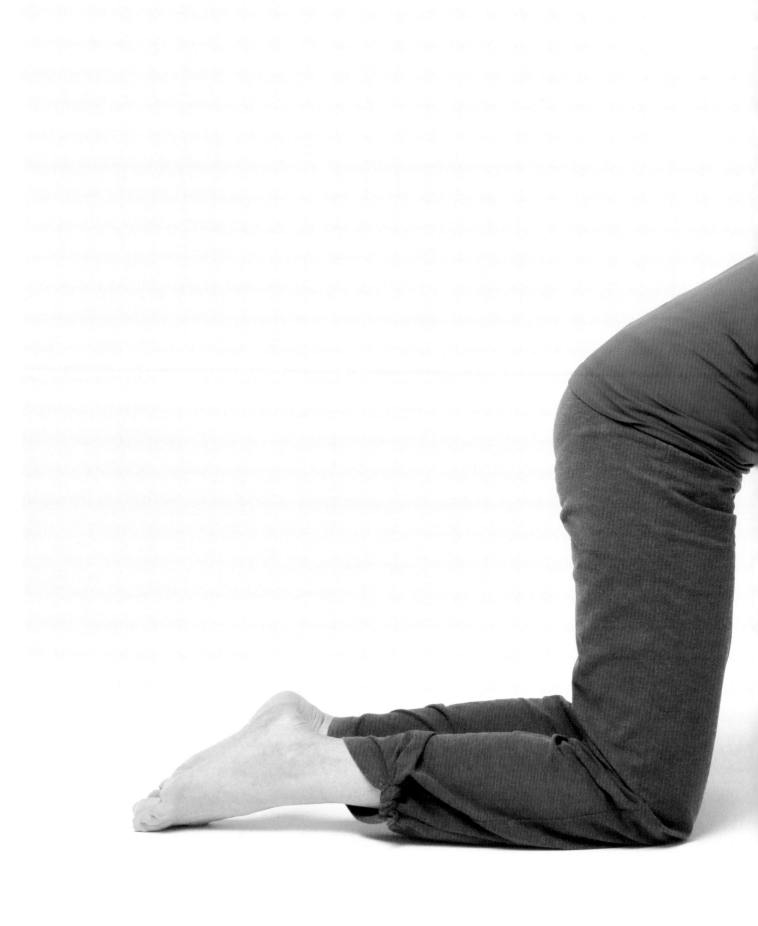

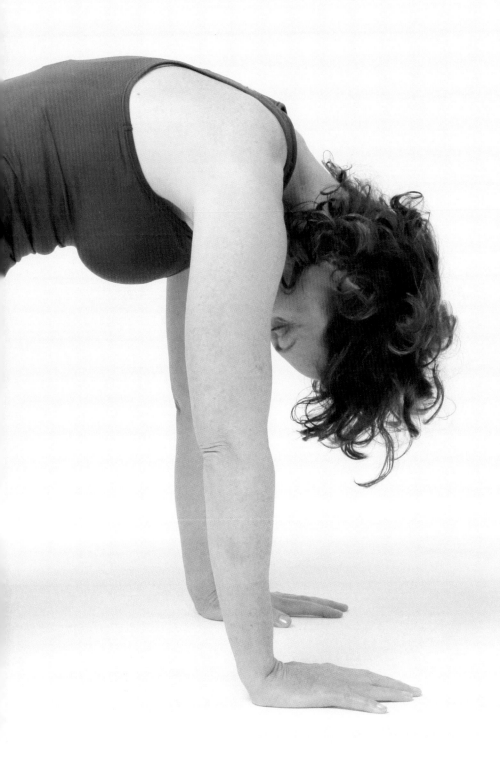

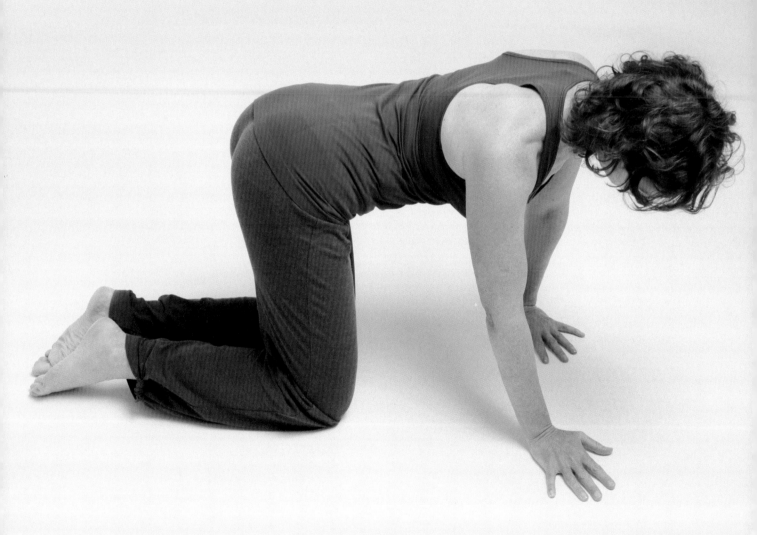

FUNCTIONAL ASANAS: SIDE BENDS

As I explained in chapter one, the bulk of yoga asanas that I practise are based around functional movement – that is, movements for which human beings are anatomically well adapted and for which we have developed a resilience over our evolutionary history. The human spine has been used to repeatedly side bend, flex, extend and rotate as part of locomotion and in daily life, and the nervous system has thus developed an understanding of these movements. These asanas are therefore likely to be both safe and useful in our yoga practice, which is why they form a large part of this book.

Side-bending is rarely used on its own in human beings, but it is a fundamental aspect of many other movements we make. It is integral to the creeping–crawling movements that babies employ before standing, and this is carried over into running and walking. It may not be obvious, but every time you lift your feet off the floor in locomotion, the spine side-bends. This is particularly significant in the lower spine, as it is the side-bending of the lumbar spine that causes the rotation of the pelvis when we walk, providing the 'engine' for locomotion. (Serge Gracovetsky's book *The Spinal Engine* gives a detailed explanation of this, for those of a scientific orientation.)

We also side-bend when we bend forward to lift things that are not directly in front of us. This is particularly clear if we are using a shovel, where the spine has to flex, side-bend and rotate in one movement.

When we lean back to get something from the back seat of the car (when sitting in the front seat) side-bending and rotation are performed together.

Essentially, the more clearly mapped we become in our bodies when it comes to the primary patterns of spinal movement – flexion, extension, rotation and side-bending – the better equipped we are for the combined movements.

IN THIS SECTION

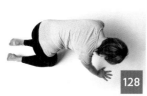 128
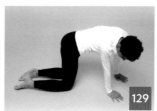 129
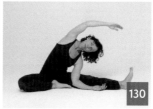 130
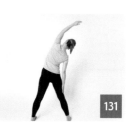 131

ALL-FOURS SIDE BEND

PURPOSE
To find out how well-mapped/compliant your body is for side-bending, and to slowly improve it through attentive practice.

APPROACHING THE ASANA
1. Come onto all fours and find the appropriate support through your shoulders and lumbar spine, by noticing where the hands need to go to give you the best feeling of support. You may need to experiment a little, sinking and pushing a little through the shoulders to start with so that you 'find' your shoulders. Similarly, with the pelvis it may be helpful to momentarily allow the lumbar spine to sag a bit then arch up a bit until you find a place that feels like good support.
2. Imagine you have a tail, and then gently 'wag' it to the left and then to the right. This should have the effect of taking the spine into side-bending.

3. Settle back to the neutral mid-line and try from the other end of your torso – so, bringing your right ear towards your right hip and your left ear to the left hip. Again, this should invite the spine and the shoulders into side-bending.

SENSE OF ENQUIRY
• When 'wagging your tail', how much of your spine, shoulders and neck participate in the movement?
• Are you 'wagging your tail' or moving your pelvis from side to side?
• When taking your ear to your shoulder, are you actually doing that, or are you taking your shoulder to your ear?
• When taking your ear to shoulder, is your head side-bending or rotating?
• When taking your ear to your shoulder, how much of your spine/pelvis participates in the movement? Really try to observe and feel.

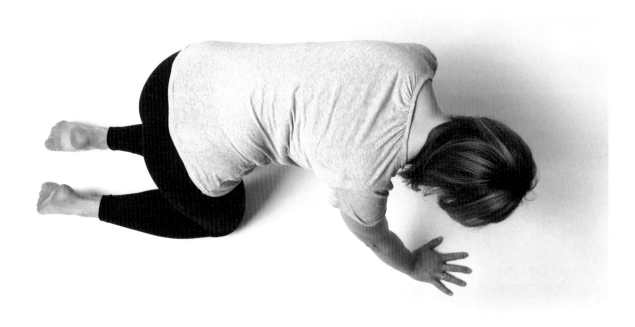

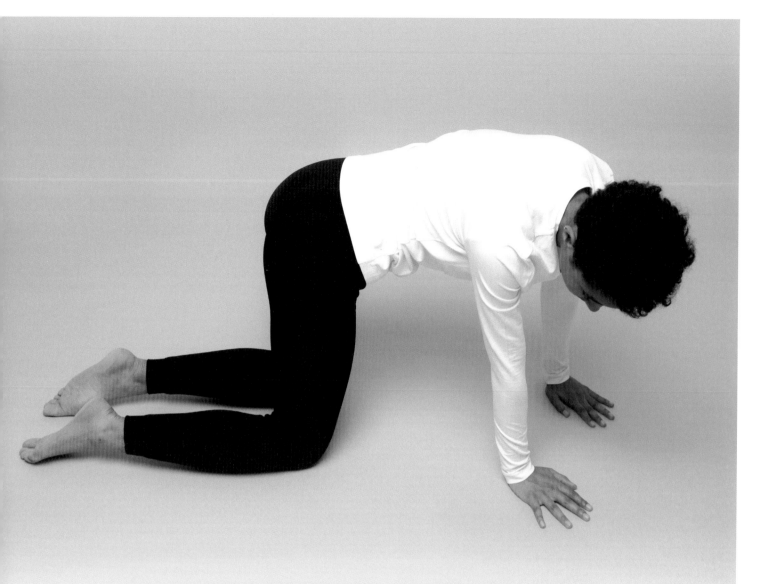

ALL-FOURS SIDE BEND, TURNING HANDS

PURPOSE
To help notice and improve the compliance/mapping of the body, particularly of the shoulder girdle in relationship to the movement of the arms. Because this is quite a subtle response of the spine, it requires us to tune in at a deep level.

APPROACHING THE ASANA
1. Come onto all fours and find the appropriate support through your shoulders and lumbar spine. Do this by noticing where the hands need to go to give you the best feeling of support. You may need to experiment a little by sinking and pushing through the shoulders (p.114) to start with so you 'find' your shoulders. Similarly, with the pelvis it may be helpful to momentarily allow the lumbar spine to sag a bit, then arch up a bit until you find a place that feels like good support.
2. Turn both your hands anti-clockwise as far as you comfortably can without strain. As you turn the hands, make sure they stay roughly under your shoulders.
3. Repeat the action, this time clockwise.

SENSE OF ENQUIRY
• As you turn your hands, do the shoulders, spine and pelvis participate usefully in the movement? Try to imagine your shoulders and spine are following the movements of the arms rather than resisting them.

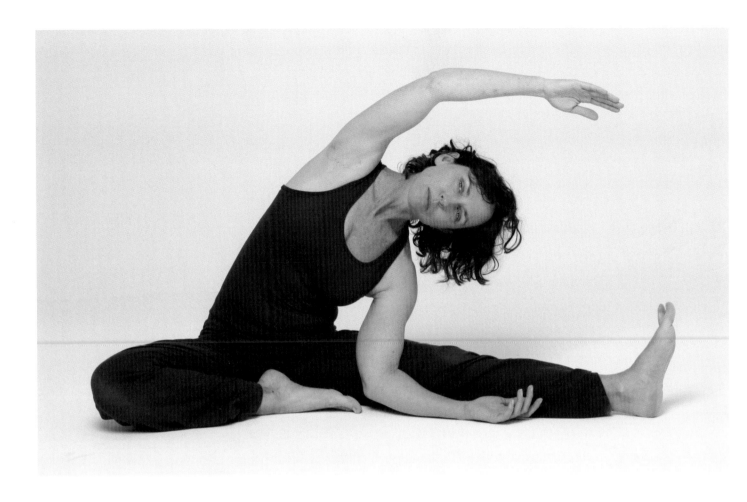

SEATED SIDE BEND

Parivrtta Janusirsasana

PURPOSE
- To help organise the legs for sitting on the floor in daily life.
- To help map the shoulders and spine for side-bending.

APPROACHING THE ASANA
1. Sit on the floor with the legs out in front of you and fold the right knee so that the sole of the right foot rests against the inside of the right thigh. Have the left leg out straight.
2. Widen the distance between the legs as far as is comfortably possible. Keep the right foot close to the inside of the left thigh.
3. Turn the body to face over the bent right leg – or however far you can get that feels comfortable. If your body can turn comfortably to face towards the bent leg, then start to bring the left ear towards the left mid thigh, allowing the movement to travel through your spine. Rest your left hand on the floor on the inside of your left knee, your right hand on the floor near your right hip.
4. Bring the head back up and repeat smoothly four or five times. Then repeat on the other side.

SENSE OF ENQUIRY
- Does the right shoulder come forward as you side-bend to the left?
- Does the weight through the sitting bones change much as you side-bend?
- Do the legs stay in place as you side bend?
- Does the trunk inadvertently move into forward-bending as you go through the side bend.

STANDING SIDE BEND

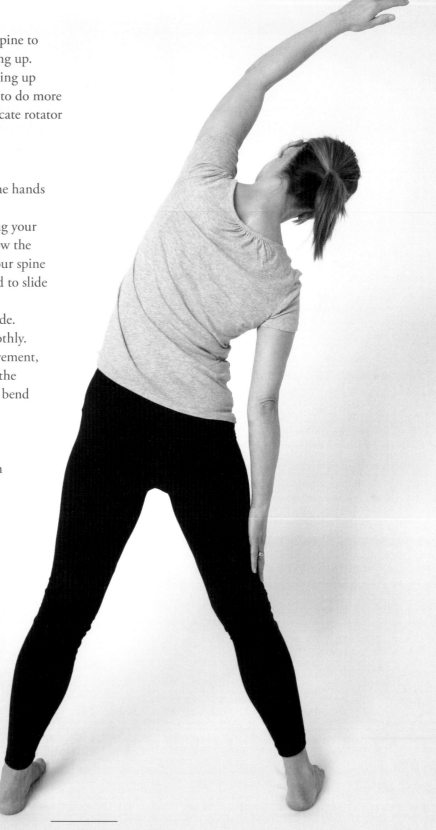

PURPOSE

To help improve the compliance of the spine to side-bending – particularly when reaching up. If the spine does not participate in reaching up movements, the shoulder girdle is asked to do more work, which can risk damage to the delicate rotator cuff muscles.

APPROACHING THE ASANA

1. Stand with the feet fairly wide and the hands resting by your side.
2. Keep looking forwards and then bring your right ear towards your right hip. Allow the movement to travel easily through your spine and shoulder, allowing the right hand to slide down the right thigh.
3. Then do the same thing on the left side. Go from side to side slowly and smoothly.
4. When you feel familiar with the movement, reach the left arm up as you bend to the right and the right arm up when you bend to the left.

SENSE OF ENQUIRY

- Notice how the weight shifts through the feet as you go through the movement.
- How smooth and fluid can you make the movement?
- Having the legs wider emphasises the movement of the spine. If you bring the feet closer together the pelvis will become more involved. So, depending on where you decide to place your focus, you can have the legs closer or wider.
- When you involve the arms, notice how the shoulder blade and collarbones become involved.

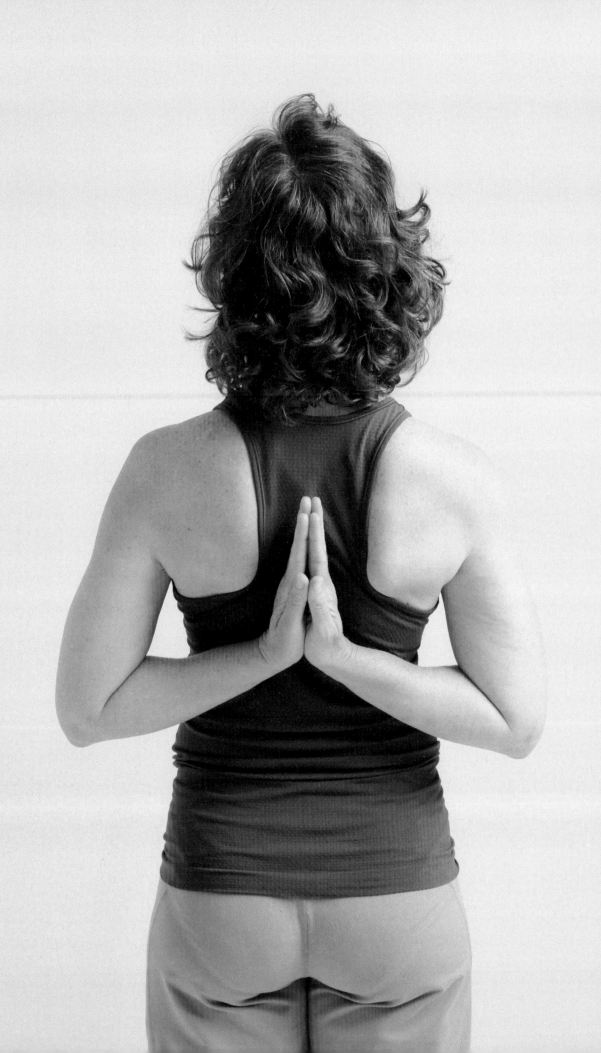

FUNCTIONAL ASANAS: EXTENSION

Although back bends are a common sight in yoga classes, they are not common in daily life. As bipeds, the need for extension is fairly limited. Even our ancestors probably only needed this movement for throwing stones or spears and climbing rock faces. The amount of extension needed for such movements is relatively small, but it is significant.

Although we are born in flexion, with no initial extension in our spines, by the time we are about a year old most of us have a well-developed lordosis in our lumbar and cervical spine. These curves in our lower and upper back distinguish us from our primate relatives who have straight spines. It seems that these curves play a significant part in our bipedal gait – a theory developed in detail by Serge Gracovetsky in *The Spinal Engine*. Because of their curves, both the lumbar and cervical spine extend easily, whilst the thoracic spine and the hip joint are better organised for flexion and are limited in their ability to extend. The thoracic spine is restricted both by the rib cage and the long spinous processes (the bony projections at the back of the vertebrae) that slope downward in the thoracic spine. The hip joint is restricted mainly by the illiofemoral ligament. If our lives become more sedentary, these areas tend to become forgotten because we can get enough movement from the neck and lumbar spine for most daily movements. However, this can lead to a situation where moving from the neck becomes increasingly familiar, and the thoracic spine and hip become less and less included when we do want to extend. Therefore, the focus of our back bends should not be how deeply we can back-bend but rather how to include the upper back and pelvis.

It is also worth pointing out that people vary hugely in terms of ability to do deep back bends. Upper spine extension abilities vary very little from person to person (by around one to four degrees), and the problem for many people here is to simply get the thoracic spine out of flexion. There is a large variation in people, however, when it comes to the lower back. This is partly due to variability in the extensibility of connective tissue, but more to do with the relative thickness of the lumbar discs compared to that of the vertebrae. If the discs are relatively thick, there is more room for extension. The deep back bends of a contortionist or very flexible yogi come from the lumbar spine. The ability to extend in this way is not particularly helpful in daily life, and a potential problem that results from us giving deep back bends value is that it can encourage people without the facility in their spines to aspire to do them – and in doing so, risk injuring themselves.

IN THIS SECTION

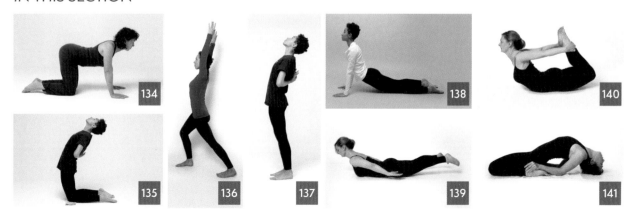

ALL-FOURS EXTENSION
(ARCHING CAT, OR COW)
Bitilasana

PURPOSE

- To help improve the 'mapping' and compliance of the spine and pelvis in extension, particularly the upper spine. It can be, and often is, combined with the flexion version (p.144) in the Cat–Cow sequence.

APPROACHING THE ASANA

1. Come onto all fours, with the hands roughly under your shoulders and knees under your hips. Find a clear contact with the floor through your hands; imagine your handprints. Then find the appropriate support through the shoulder girdle and lumbar spine. Do this by playing around a little with the sinking–pushing feelings through the shoulder girdle and tilting the pelvis up and down a bit. Once you have done that, settle into what 'feels' okay, rather than what you 'think' is straight.

2. Then take your gaze forwards and up as though you are trying to follow the movement of something that moved directly forwards and away from you and then up the wall in front

'Imagine your neck starts between your shoulder blades, rather like it does on a horse.'

---

of you. Keep your arms straight but not stiff. Imagine your neck starts between your shoulder blades, rather like it does on a horse, and think about looking up from there.

3. Repeat this movement slowly and smoothly several times, combining with the flexion version (p.144) if you like.

SENSE OF ENQUIRY

- How much of your spine and pelvis are involved in the movement?
- If you have noticed the pelvis moving, how early or late in the movement does it get involved?
- How smooth and fluid can you make the movement feel?

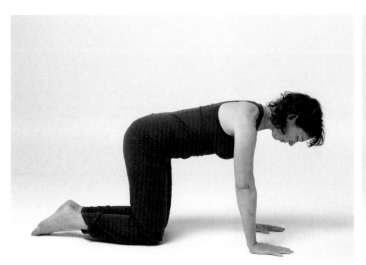
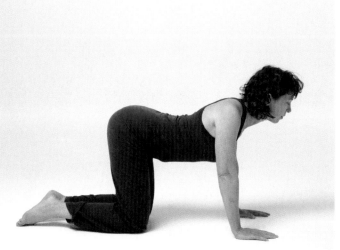

KNEELING BACK BEND
(CAMEL)
Ustrasana

———

When we are on all fours and move into extension, the pelvis moves into an anterior tilt (where the tailbone moves up towards the ceiling). This is the sensible, compliant way for the pelvis to move in this posture. It is sometimes called the *quadrupedal* or *infantile* pattern of extension. Things change, though, when we come upright onto two legs. By pushing down through the feet, the hip extensors get involved and extend the hip joint. So then, when we extend by looking up, for example, the hips will swing forwards rather than tilt anteriorly. This is the *bipedal* form of extension. However, some people carry the infantile pattern into their standing organisation and the pelvis anteriorly tilts rather than swings forward. This is very unhelpful and tends to cause a lot of compression in the lower back in standing back bends.

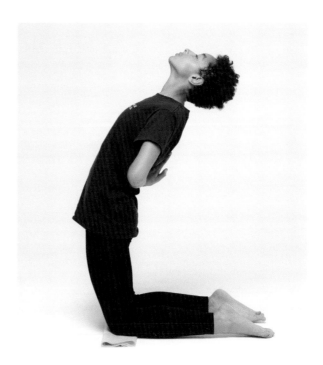

PURPOSE

To help map the movement of extension throughout the body, especially the hips. In this back bend, the hip joints are more naturally constrained in extension by the tension created by the quadriceps, which, in this position, are lengthened over the knee. Finding this extension pattern in the hips, through practising this asana regularly, will make the standing extension pose feel considerably easier, because in standing the constraint of the quadriceps is removed.

APPROACHING THE ASANA

1. Start by kneeling up and with the arms relaxed and hanging beside your torso. You can tuck the toes under if it helps you to feel more stable.
2. Remind yourself that, muscularly, the neck starts between your shoulder blades, and then take your gaze forwards and up towards the ceiling. Allow your shoulders and arms to relax and fall back as you look up, just as far as is comfortable. Then bring your gaze back to the horizontal.
3. Repeat this fairly slowly several times. As you look up, allow the hips to swing forwards. When this feels easy and familiar, tuck your toes under, so that you come into the hinges of the toes, and when you look up take your gaze a little further up and back. Some people may be able to reach back and touch their heels at the end of the movement… but do not go searching for them! However, if you can get your hands *comfortably* to your feet, allow your eyes to look back just a little.
4. Repeat this several times until your whole body starts to feel familiar with the movement.

SENSE OF ENQUIRY

- What happens to your pelvis as you look up? Does it swing forwards or does it tend to anteriorly rotate (so that your bottom sticks out)?
- What happens to your breastbone as you look up? Does it tend to rise or does it sink?
- What happens to your breathing as you look up? Does it remain reasonably easy or does it start to feel strained? If the latter, can you notice when and where the strain is felt?
- How far you look up will vary from person to person. Never go further than feels comfortable and do not allow a sense of strain to develop at the front of the neck.

———

STANDING BACK BEND
(WARRIOR ONE)
Virabhadrasana I

This is a very common action in daily life; every time we look or reach up we extend our body. It is not uncommon, though, to find people only extending with the neck or lower back because these areas are well mapped, while the upper spine and hip joint are not. Overuse in the well-mapped areas often causes pain through compression in the lower back and neck.

PURPOSE
To develop compliance in extension throughout the body. This practice helps integrate the hips and upper spine into extension movements in standing.

APPROACHING THE ASANA
1. Start by standing in Mountain pose (p.176) with the feet about hip width apart and roughly parallel. Pay attention to mapping the whole footprint on the floor. Relax the shoulders and arms and neck and have your gaze towards the horizon.
2. Then take your gaze upwards towards the ceiling (or sky). Remember, muscularly your neck starts between your shoulder blades, so imagine looking up from there.
3. Allow your pelvis to swing comfortably forwards as you look up. Repeat this several times until the movement feels comfortable and familiar. If you feel strain in the neck, look up less far and go less far forward with your pelvis. Keep the arms relaxed and allow the shoulder blades to slide back and slightly towards each other (do not pull them back!). Notice whether the breastbone rises or falls.
4. Take your right leg one step forwards, initially keeping it straight. Then, go through the looking-up movement again, allowing the pelvis and therefore the front knee to bend and move forward.
5. Then bring your gaze back to the horizontal and let the hip and knee return to their starting position, straightening the leg again. Repeat several times until you feel the movement of the pelvis and front knee are just part of the looking up movement.
6. The next time you perform the movement, reach up with the arms as you look up, imagining that you are trying to catch a beach ball that is almost out of reach as it passes over your head. Then repeat on other side.

SENSE OF ENQUIRY
- Do the knee and pelvis swing forwards easily as you look up? Simply notice what is happening. If the pelvis feels reluctant to move, be patient; do not force the issue but instead bring your awareness to the front of the hips as you look up, and as best you can simply 'allow' the movement to develop. Note that it can sometimes take many months to integrate poorly mapped areas into a movement.
- Does the breastbone rise or fall as you look up?
- Do you feel steady and stable throughout the movement?
- Does your breathing feel easy and comfortable throughout the movement?

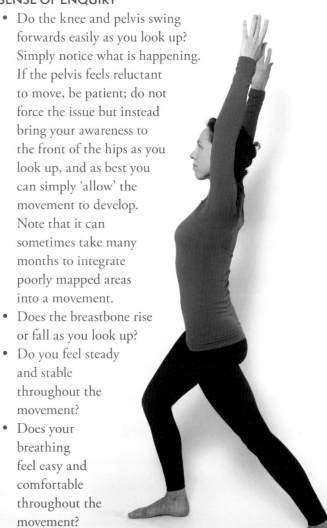

STANDING BACK BEND
WITH ARMS IN REVERSE PRAYER

PURPOSE

- To more explicitly help map the movement of extension throughout the body, especially the upper back and shoulder blades.
- To help map the relationship between the scapulae and spine by noticing how the hands open and close in the movement, as the spine moves from flexion to extension.

APPROACHING THE ASANA

1. Stand in Mountain (p.176) with the feet about hip width apart and roughly parallel. Pay attention to mapping the whole footprint on the floor. Relax the shoulders and arms and neck and direct your gaze towards the horizon.

2. Then bring the hands into prayer behind you, relax the arms and allow the elbows to drop. For some people this movement will be too painful, and it is certainly not worth trying to force your arm into this position. If this is the case, it is more useful to do some of the all fours shoulder work (see p.114).

3. Allow the head to drop forwards and let the upper body slump. Then slowly bring the head back up and go into slight extension by bringing the gaze up (it can be useful to remember that in the muscular sense your neck starts between your shoulders). Allow the shoulders to follow the movement of the spine. Repeat this action a few times, going from a little flexion to a little extension, just far enough that you can feel the shoulders and arms follow the movement.

4. Start to feel the way the shoulders respond to the movement of the spine. As you move into extension, imagine your spine arching over your hands. You can then very slightly exaggerate the movement of the arms and hands as you go through the movement.

SENSE OF ENQUIRY

- Notice the movement of the shoulder blades, breastbone and pelvis as you move from flexion to extension. Which way do the shoulders move when you bend forwards and when you bend backwards? How easily does the breastbone sink when you flex, and rise when you extend? And does the pelvis move back easily in flexion and shift forwards in extension?
- Do you notice the hands opening and closing with the movement?

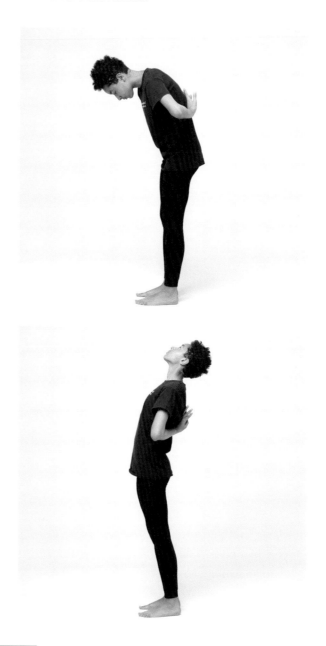

UPWARD-FACING DOG AND COBRA

Urdhva Mukha Svanasana and Bhujangasana

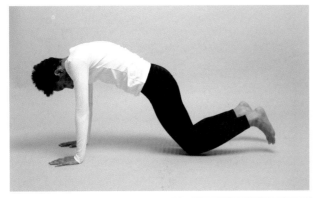

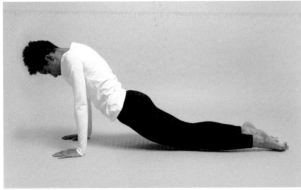

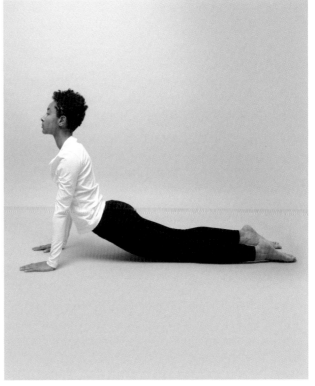

In Upward-facing Dog the pelvis is off the ground, while in Cobra it stays on the ground. However, though these poses are often treated as separate postures within yoga practice, there is little difference between them when approached with the aim of mapping extension. It is thus best to simply leave the pelvis where it feels most comfortable.

PURPOSE

To help map the movement of extension throughout the body, particularly the upper spine and neck.

APPROACHING THE ASANA

1. Come onto all fours and take your hands a good hand's length further forward from their starting position. Find the appropriate support through the shoulders, arms and hands by first sinking and pushing a little through the shoulders and settling on something that feels useful.

2. Swing the body forwards so that the legs straighten, and allow the pelvis to drop towards the floor. Reassess the support through your shoulders to make sure it still feels appropriate.

3. Bring the gaze up to just above the horizon. Remember that the muscles of your neck start between your shoulder blades, and thus so should your gaze. Only stay a few moments and then come back onto all fours.

4. Repeat slowly and smoothly a few times. If you feel compression in the lower back, try a variation on your elbows (Sphinx), rather than trying to solve it by tucking the tailbone down.

SENSE OF ENQUIRY

- Did you stiffen or collapse through the shoulders when you moved into the back bend?
- Did you feel the pelvis move forwards a little as you brought the gaze up? Simply try to notice.

PRONE BACK BEND
Salabhasana

PURPOSE

To help map the pattern of extension throughout the body. In this movement we are asking the whole body to extend against gravity. It requires real attention to make this movement feel comfortable.

APPROACHING THE ASANA

1. Start by lying on your tummy with your arms beside your torso and the palms facing down, if that feels comfortable. (You might be more comfortable with a folded blanket under your pelvis.) Rest your forehead on the floor.

2. Start to lift your head a little off the floor. And take your gaze to about a metre or two in front of you. As with most of the postures in this section, it is useful to remember that your neck muscles start from between your shoulder blades, and so to imagine you are lifting your head from here.

3. Lift your arms from the floor, remembering to include the shoulders. Notice if you have a

tendency to draw the shoulders towards your ears as you lift them.

4. Then bring your legs a little off the floor as well. If you find you get a feeling of compression in your lower back, try starting by lifting your legs first and then the head.

5. If you find the lower back feels compressed in this movement, try lifting the legs first, which usually helps a lot.

SENSE OF ENQUIRY

- When you lift you head is it your tummy or pelvis that presses into the floor? This movement is sometimes done with the infantile pattern of extension mapped into the pelvis (see explanation on p.135, Kneeling Back Bend).

- Do you feel any compression in your lower back? If so, do not come up so high. Or as explained above, try lifting the legs first.

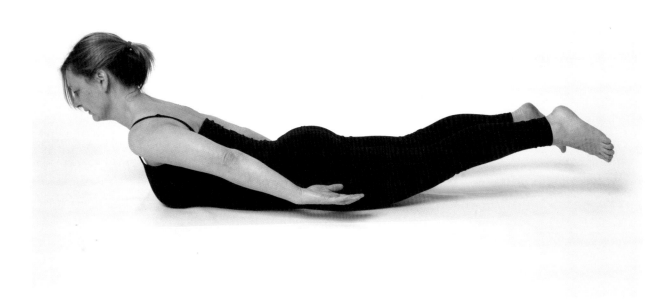

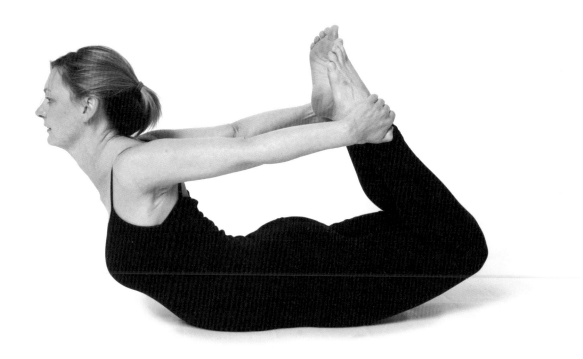

HANDS-TO-ANKLE PRONE BACK BEND
(BOW)

Dhanurasana

PURPOSE

- To help map the upper spine and neck in extension, through a movement that exaggerates the action of the shoulder blades.
- To help find extension at the hips as part of the whole body extension pattern.

APPROACHING THE ASANA

1. Start by lying on your tummy and resting your forehead on the floor. Give yourself time to relax in this position.
2. Bend your knees and take hold of your ankles with your hands. Bring your head off the floor and take your gaze a few metres in front of you.
3. Pull your ankles away from your hips so that the arms and shoulders are drawn back and the upper back is pulled more into extension. Do not pull with your arms! Lift your knees a little off the floor.
4. Lower yourself down and repeat a few times, trying to make the movement smoother and more fluid each time.

SENSE OF ENQUIRY

- Notice whether you are using the legs at all to pull the arms back or if you are pulling on your ankles with your arms.
- Notice whether you can keep your breathing appropriate to the effort required, or whether it becomes ragged with periods of holding.

KNEELING SUPINE BACK BEND
(FISH POSE VARIATION)
Paryankasana

This is a fairly advanced posture and you should be able to do a comfortable Hero pose (p.166) before you attempt it. It is also not worth trying if you are fairly rounded in the upper back, as most of the movement will then likely come from the neck, thereby risking compressing the area at the base of the skull.

PURPOSE
The weight of the head coming back can be very useful in getting us to map the upper thoracic spine, which is encouraged to move into extension here. However, it is important not to pull the head back and compress the back of the neck.

APPROACHING THE ASANA
1. Start by sitting in Hero (p.166) and bring the heel of your hands to just behind your toes. Rest your fingers, facing forwards, on the soles of your feet.
2. Rest back onto your elbows and then start to bring your head back. At the same time, move your elbows forwards enough so that you can bring the crown of the head to the floor. At least two thirds of the weight should come through the arms, and about a third on the head.
3. Again, think of your neck starting between your shoulders as you bring it back to the floor. Push down into your elbows and hands to come back into Hero. Only stay a moment or two before returning to Hero. If it feels reasonably comfortable, repeat it three or four times.

SENSE OF ENQUIRY
- As you draw your head back, allow the breastbone to follow the extension movement.
- Be sure you do not poke your chin up and compress the back of the neck.
- Allow the front of the pelvis to tip forwards. Do not try to 'tuck' the tailbone under.
- Do you feel comfortable at the base of the skull?

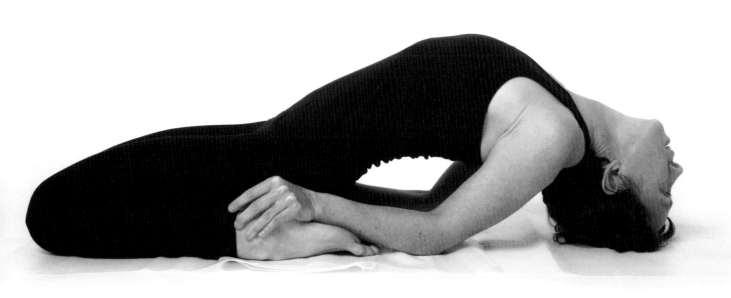

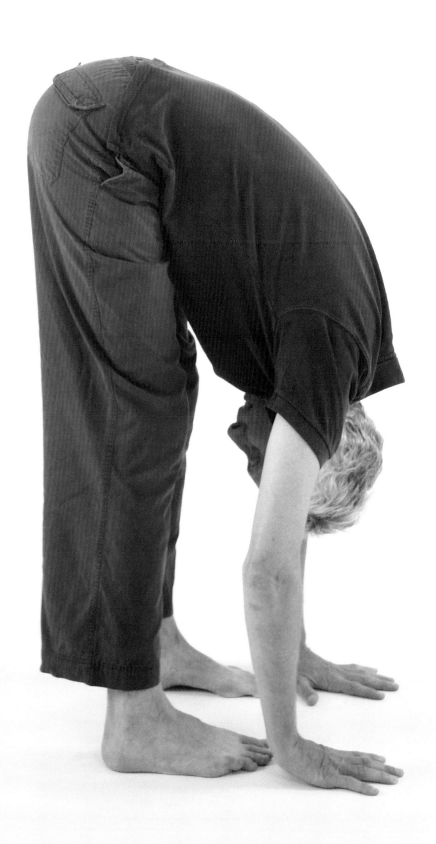

FUNCTIONAL ASANAS: FLEXION

There is a lot of controversy in yoga about the best way to bend forward. Should we do it with a straight spine or a rounded spine? Should the knees be straight or bent? Each view is shored up with examples of why this view is right and the others wrong.

Much of this discussion stems from a 1980s dispute between two Canadians: professor of spine biomechanics Stuart McGill and mathematician Serge Gracovetsky. McGill argued that repeated bending of the spine caused degradation of the discs and that therefore it was important to keep the spine straight when bending forwards. Gracovetsky argued that if you do not bend your back, you cannot utilise the lumbodorsal fascia; but if you bend forwards with the spine flexed, the lumbodorsal fascia is stretched out to its maximum length and can then be used by the gluteal muscles to transmit their power to the spine and take the load of the upper body. He also took a more anthropological perspective, noting that people all around the world often did round their backs when bending down, and that children did often. His has always seemed to me to be a much more compelling argument than McGill's. In the end, of course, we should pick things up, lift things and bend forwards in the way that feels most comfortable. What Gracovetsky is taking issue with is the much-repeated edict that it is dangerous to flex the spine. He was not arguing that you *have* to bend the spine.

Much of our nervousness about teaching flexion is based on the fact that, in modern societies, many of us spend a great deal of time in flexion – particularly those who work at a desk all day. So, why should we flex it more? I have dealt with this issue in the section on body mapping, but, in brief, if we want to free ourselves of constraining postures, we need to help the nervous system 'understand' how it arrived at the situation it is in – and then retrain it. The best way to do that is to open up the whole repertoire of flexion available to the body, and to be able to sense how this feels, so that we know how to change when we need to. This is a much better strategy than simply telling people to sit or stand up straight.

IN THIS SECTION

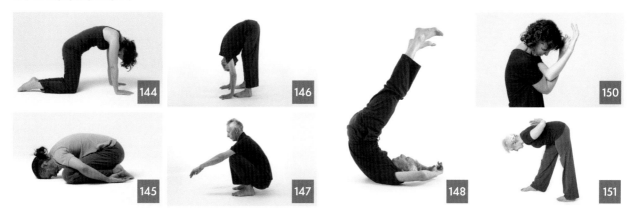

143

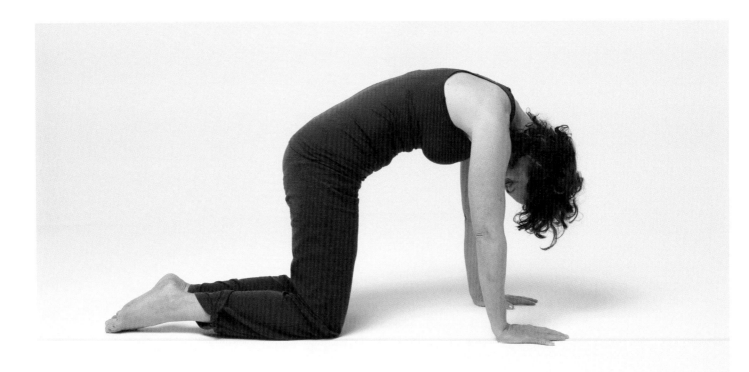

ALL-FOURS FORWARD BEND
(CAT)

Marjaryasana

PURPOSE

This is often paired with the all fours extension movement (aka Cow; p.134). It is useful to move from one to the other, to experience and map a whole pattern of movement in the spine from maximum flexion to maximum extension. Here I will look at the flexion part of the movement.

APPROACHING THE ASANA

1. Come onto all fours and find the appropriate support through the shoulder girdle and lumbar spine. You can find the appropriate support by firstly allowing the rib cage to slowly sink through the shoulder girdle, and then doing the opposite, pushing it away from the floor. Then, tuck the tailbone under a little, and then go the other way, sending it towards the ceiling. Go quietly through these small movements a few times until you settle on an all-fours position that feels appropriate to you rather than one you think you should be in. Soften your neck.

2. Look down at the floor directly below you, and slowly take your gaze through your knees and imagine looking through the knees and at the wall behind you. Look as far up the wall as you comfortably can. Keep the arms straight but not stiff. Return the gaze to its starting point, looking forward.

3. Repeat this movement slowly and smoothly several times.

SENSE OF ENQUIRY

When you bring your gaze either up or down, notice if and when the pelvis becomes involved in the action. Try not to artificially move the pelvis. Instead, if it does not move, try to sense what you are doing to prevent it moving. In the end, we are looking for the pelvis to move almost the moment that the head starts to move.

CHILD'S POSE

Pindasana

PURPOSE

- To practise putting the ankles, knees and hips through a normal range of movement.
- To help us look for comfort in a simple movement.
- To allow the spine to fold forwards in a comfortable position.

APPROACHING THE ASANA

1. Start by sitting upright on your heels, and feel the weight of your body on your feet. If your knees feel uncomfortable, put a folded blanket or a block between your pelvis and lower legs and sit on that. If you feel pressure on your feet from the floor, roll up a slim blanket and place the roll under your ankles. Be sure to have enough support to allow yourself to feel comfortable.
2. Fold forwards from your hips, until your torso is resting on your thighs. If the pressure on your abdomen is uncomfortable, widen the knees until you feel okay.
3. Decide whether it feels easier with the arms resting forwards in front of you, palms down and elbows slightly bent, or back alongside your waist with your palms turned up. You can stay in the pose for as long as it feels comfortable.

SENSE OF ENQUIRY

- Do your knees, ankles and feet feel comfortable?
- Does your breathing feel easy? Be curious.
- Is there any way you could make yourself more comfortable anywhere in your body?
- Let the weight fall through the points of contact to the ground. So, if your head rests on the floor, really let it rest and feel heavy. Let your arms rest on the floor. Allow your trunk to rest on your thighs.

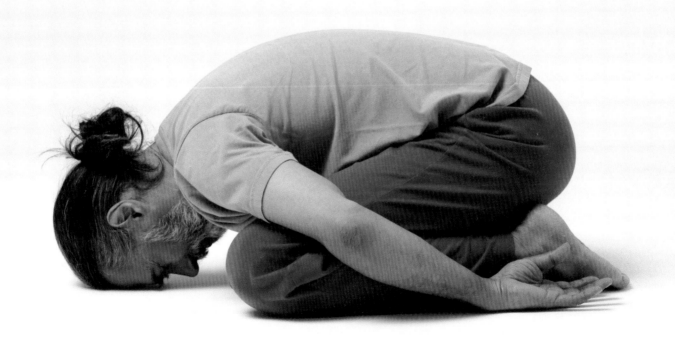

STANDING FORWARD BEND

Uttanasana

As mentioned in the chapter introduction, I take the view that bending forwards and rolling down is fine. However, all movements need to be mitigated by feelings of pain and discomfort. If you have a current disc problem or a back spasm, a standing forward bend might well be painful, and the all-fours variation (Cat; p.144) may be more helpful.

PURPOSE
- To allow the whole of the spine to be in flexion.
- To decompress the lumbar discs.

APPROACHING THE ASANA
1. Come into standing with the feet hip-width apart and roughly parallel, and arms by your sides.
2. Allow the chin to relax down, relax the shoulders, and slowly roll all the way down to the floor, letting the arms hang heavy.
3. Let the knees soften as you roll down. If your hamstrings are very tight, let the knees bend as much as you need to reduce the feeling of strain at the back of the legs.
4. Try to 'reverse the film' on the way back into standing.

SENSE OF ENQUIRY
- When you begin the movement, what happens to the shoulder blades, the breastbone and the pelvis? Try to really pay attention.
- How is the distribution of weight between your inner and outer footprints?
- Can you manage to keep your arms and shoulders relaxed throughout?

'Slowly roll all the way down to the floor, letting the arms hang heavy.'

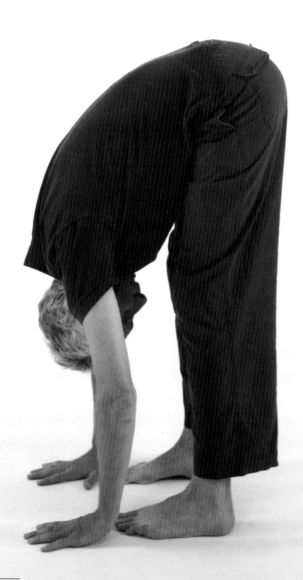

SQUATTING

The practice of squatting can help us notice tension that often accrues in the groin and lower back. In daily movement, we often need to look up when we squat, which introduces an element of extension and therefore activity in the hip flexors. (See pp.58–60 for an explanation of how extension of the head and upper back is accompanied by anterior tilting of the pelvis.) So I want to draw attention to the possibility that we might have maintained tightness in the groin even when we do not need it – i.e. when looking down.

It is important to try to keep the neck relaxed throughout if we want to bring release into the hip flexors.

PURPOSE
- To put the knees and hips through their full range of flexion.
- To improve or maintain the range of dorsiflexion at the ankle.
- To allow the lumbar spine some decompression.
- To relax the hip and neck flexors in a situation where they often unconsciously contract.

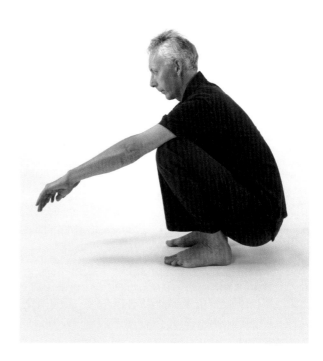

APPROACHING THE ASANA
1. Start standing up with feet hip-width apart and parallel, and allow the body to softly roll into a forward bend (a 'rag doll' forward bend).
2. Keep the neck relaxed and start to bend the knees towards a squatting position. Keep the whole body relaxed the whole time. If you find the heels need to lift off the ground that is fine. But even if your heels lift off, keep some attention on the balance between the inner and outer foot. Let the pelvis really drop. Relax the neck and the shoulders.
3. Then slowly straighten the legs back into a forward bend.
4. Repeat the whole movement slowly a few times, each time trying to keep the body softer and more relaxed throughout.

5. From time to time when you are practising squatting, simply come onto your haunches, resting your pelvis on your heels and your elbows on your thighs. Relax your neck and look down, while swinging your knees very gently from side to side.

SENSE OF ENQUIRY
- Can you manage to keep your neck and shoulders relaxed throughout the movement?
- Do you tighten up in the groin as you move into the squat?
- Do you manage to keep some balance through the inner and outer foot as you go through the movement?

SPINAL ROLLING AND SHOULDER STAND

PURPOSE

- To map the pattern of flexion throughout the body.
- To relax the muscles of extension – particularly the neck extensors and the lumbar extensors – through reciprocal inhibition (the process whereby the muscles on one side of a joint relax to accomodate the contraction of the muscles on the other side).

APPROACHING THE ASANA

1. Start by sitting with the knees bent and feet on the floor in front of you. Bring your gaze down, as though you were looking at your navel, and let the breastbone sink.
2. Reach forwards with the arms and shoulders and slowly roll backwards, keeping a sense of curling in your spine. Resist throwing yourself back.
3. Bring your knees in and reach your legs over your head towards the floor. How much you need to straighten your legs for your toes to move towards the ground will depend a bit on the proportion of your leg length to body length.
4. Then 'rewind the film' back to your starting position. Imagine you are trying to keep your spine like a wheel as you roll.
5. If you find this difficult, either speed the movement up a little (not too fast!) or use your hands and arms to help you roll over, but still try to maintain the curled shape.

SENSE OF ENQUIRY

- Did you manage to keep looking towards your navel throughout the movement?
- If you find this fairly easy, try slowing the movement down.
- Where are you breathing?

SHOULDER STAND VARIATION

I am not a fan of the traditional shoulder stand. Rather, I see this asana as a natural development from spinal rolling. To be able to arrive in any sort of shoulder stand position you need to go through spinal rolling first. If you cannot do this, the only way into a shoulder stand is to heave yourself up with your arms –and this implies that the body is unable to support itself in this position, in which case it is an unwise thing to do. You will simply be resting all your weight on your wrists and potentially creating strain in your neck.

If, however, you are able to roll your feet over your head into a rounded plough, you can then see if it is possible to raise the legs so that the feet point more to the ceiling. See how far you can straighten up without causing strain in the neck. Whatever degree of straightness you have is what your healthy shoulder stand should be. Do not try to straighten more by pushing with the hands. Be happy with whatever banana shape you have arrived in. Do not stay here for any length of time before carefully rolling down again. Practise slowly, rolling over into plough, then lifting feet towards the ceiling. Support your pelvis with your hands when you have straightened to your comfortable limit, then pause for a few breaths and roll down slowly again.

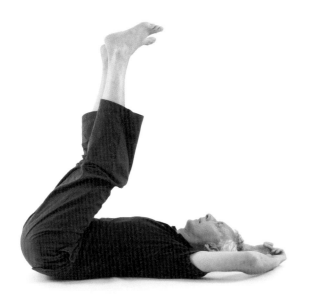

'Whatever degree of straightness you have is what your healthy shoulder stand should be. Do not try to straighten more by pushing with the hands. Be happy with whatever banana shape you have arrived in.'

——————

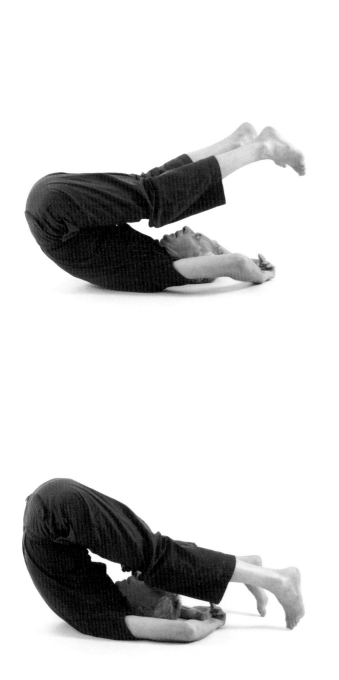

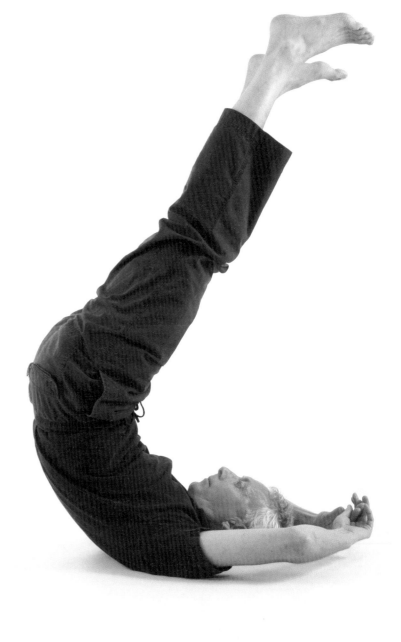

EAGLE-ARMS FORWARD BEND

Garudasana variation

───────

PURPOSE

- To map a better relationship between the movements of the shoulder blades and the movements of the spine.
- To help reduce strain for the rotator cuff muscles.

APPROACHING THE ASANA

1. Come into standing. Reach your arms forwards as if you were going to give a beach ball a gentle hug. As you reach your arms and shoulders forward, drop your chin a little and allow the breastbone to sink.

2. Bring the left arm over the right arm at the elbows, and bring the forearms to the vertical. If possible, bring the left hand back past the right hand and bring the palms together.

3. Fold the body forwards into a soft forward bend, and allow the wrists and elbows to drop towards the floor. Let the weight of your arms draw them down, though keeping them crossed. Do not actively take them towards the floor or away from you. If you feel you need to allow the knees to bend then do so. Only stay as long as is comfortable and not more than thirty seconds.

4. Come back up into standing, release the arms, and then repeat the whole movement with the right arm going over the left.

SENSE OF ENQUIRY

- Do not 'pull' on your arms; wrap them around each other loosely, not tightly. The rotator cuff muscles that run from the scapula to the top of the humerus are relatively weak.
- As you fold forward, be sure to relax your neck, allowing the head to feel heavy.

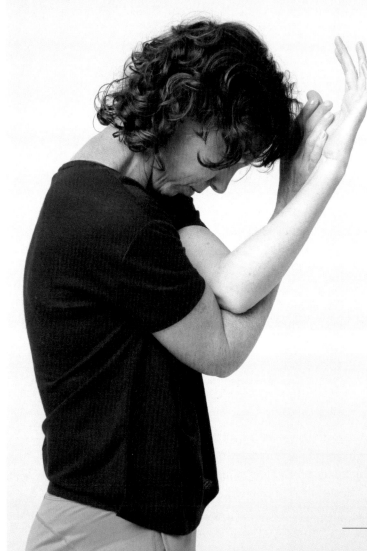

'Let the weight of your arms draw them down. Do not actively take them towards the floor or away from you. If you feel you need to allow the knees to bend then do so.'

───────

STEPPING-FORWARD FORWARD BEND

Parsvottanasana

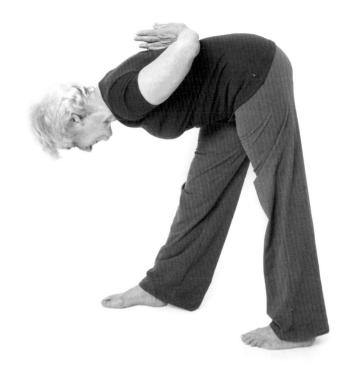

This is an interesting movement to explore what happens to the hips and the spine when we bend forwards. What we discover is that the spine and pelvis tend to respond to the direction we are looking. So, if you are looking forwards as you bend forwards, you will notice the spine straightens, and the spine and pelvis go into an extension pattern. If, on the other hand, we look down as we bend forwards, the spine and pelvis tend to move into flexion. This observation will influence what we want to do with the hands when we practise this movement.

PURPOSE

To clarify the relationship between the orientation of the head and the action of the pelvis as we bend forwards.

APPROACHING THE ASANA

1. Come into standing and take a step forwards with your right leg. Settle into your footprints, feeling the weight evenly in the inner and outer aspects of your feet. Keep your arms relaxed by your side.

2. Wait until you feel stable, then look down at your front foot and start to bend forwards keeping your legs relatively straight, if you can, until your hands touch the floor or you feel constrained by the hamstrings. Your arms stay relaxed from the shoulders.

3. Then 'rewind the film' and come back into standing.

4. Repeat the movement, but this time keep the gaze looking straight ahead, again moving until either you feel constrained by the hamstrings or your hands touch the floor. Then 'rewind the film' once more, until you are back in standing.

5. Repeat this a few times, alternating between bringing the gaze down towards your front foot and then looking straight ahead. Notice

the difference in the way the spine and pelvis respond. Repeat these movements with the left foot forwards.

6. If you want to add the arms into this movement, use the prayer position behind your back when you are looking straight ahead as you bend forwards, and the Eagle-arms position (p.150) when you are looking down at your front foot. This reduces potential strain on the rotator cuff muscles that can happen if the same arm position is used regardless of what the spine is doing.

SENSE OF ENQUIRY

- Do you feel stable and comfortable throughout the movement?
- How clearly did you notice the different action of the spine and pelvis when you changed the orientation of the head?
- Do not allow feelings of strain at the shoulder girdle. Release the arms if they feel too uncomfortable.
- Try to maintain good footprints throughout the movement.

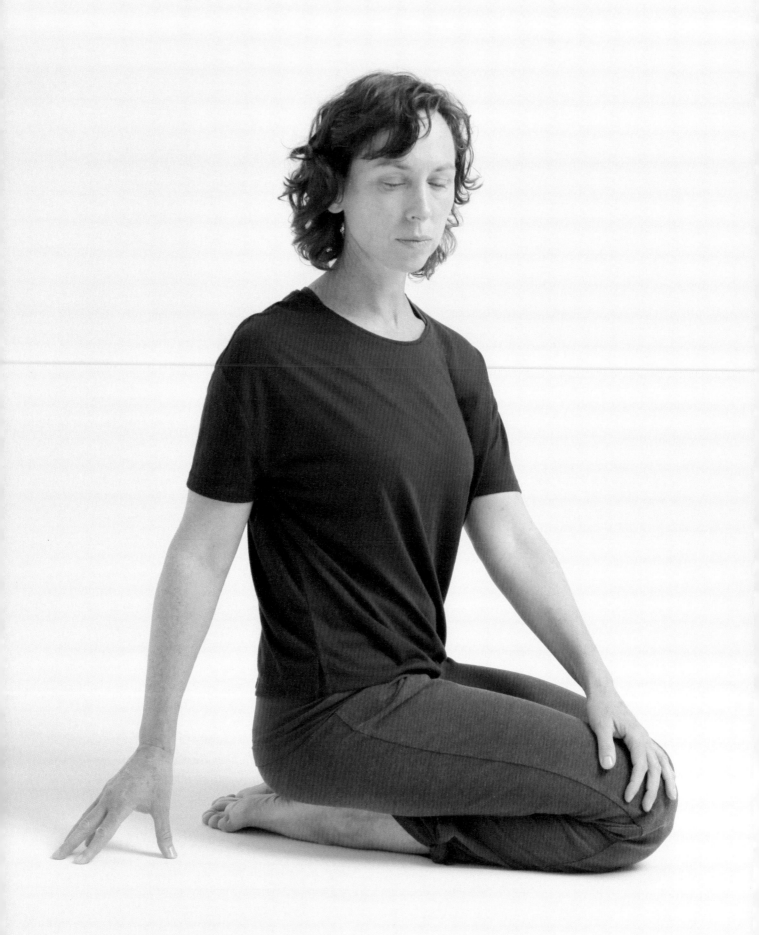

FUNCTIONAL ASANAS: ROTATION

A small but significant point: it seems to me there is a difference between the terms 'twisting' and 'turning'. With twisting, we are talking about one end of the object being twisted in one direction whilst the other end goes in the other direction. This is the sort of action you employ if you are wringing out a wet cloth. In normal life, the only time we use anything like this action is in locomotion. We notice it particularly if we are running quickly, when the left side of the pelvis will go forwards as the shoulder on that side goes back. Other than that there are no serious movements where we employ twisting. Instead, the action is actually turning. For example, we may look behind us because someone called out, and here we turn the head first and then the shoulders, chest and pelvis follow. There is rotation happening but it all goes in the same direction – unlike with twisting. So, apart from locomotion, we can consider turning functional and twisting not so functional. In yoga, I am therefore more interested in turning than twisting.

It is also useful to bear in mind when practising yoga that the amount of rotation available in the spine varies at different points. There is most availability in the cervical spine, then the thoracic, with the lumbar spine having the least. It should also be noted that more rotation becomes available in the lumbar spine if it is side-bent first, but that this is an action that may have a deleterious effect on the lumbar discs. So it is inadvisable to practise a movement that brings a strong rotation movement into an already side-bent lumbar spine, as I point out on pages 105–106.

IN THIS SECTION

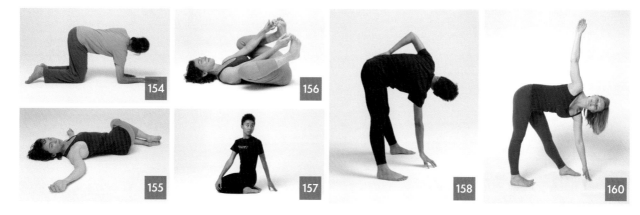

ALL-FOURS TURNING

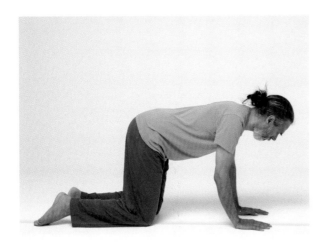

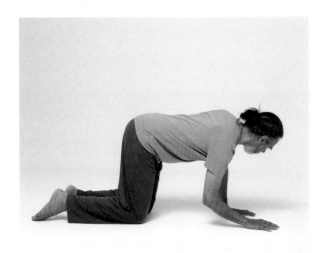

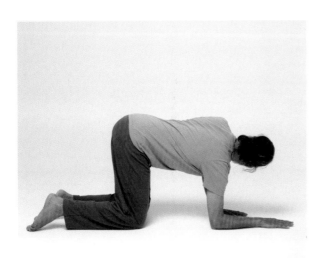

PURPOSE

To put the shoulders, rib cage and spine through a full range of rotation to the left and right sides.

APPROACHING THE ASANA

1. Come onto all fours, and find the appropriate support through the shoulder girdle and lower back (see p.114).
2. Turn your head to look to the left and then up towards the ceiling or sky. Allow the right elbow to bend and bring it to the floor roughly where your hand has been. Keep the left arm fairly straight.
3. When you have turned as far as you can comfortably go, come back onto all fours and repeat the movement to the right.
4. Go through the movement on the left and right side several times until the movement feels smooth and familiar.

SENSE OF ENQUIRY

- When you turn to the left, be careful to keep the left arm reasonably straight.
- Try to turn your head at about 90 degrees, so you are looking at right angles to your trunk, rather than looking back.
- Is the action smooth and fluid, and does your support feel steady and quiet?

'Try to turn your head at about 90 degrees, so you are looking at right angles to your trunk, rather than looking back.'

SUPINE TURNING

PURPOSE
To help develop compliance in the relationship of the shoulder to the rib cage and spine.

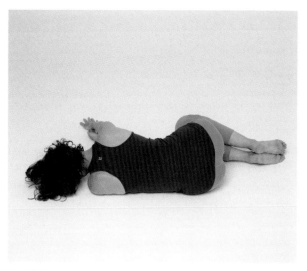

APPROACHING THE ASANA
1. Start by lying on your left side with your knees bent and your thighs at about a right angle to your trunk. Have your arms parallel to your thighs, with the right arm lying on the left. Rest your head on the floor. If that is uncomfortable, put the minimum amount of support under your head to make it comfortable, but try not to reduce the side-bending in the neck to zero. Relax yourself as much as possible in this position so that your head rests, your ribs rest, your upper leg rests and your upper arm rests.
2. Keeping a very soporific feeling in the body, slide your right hand forwards past your lower hand as far as it can comfortably go, so you are turning towards the floor. Let the rest of your body follow.

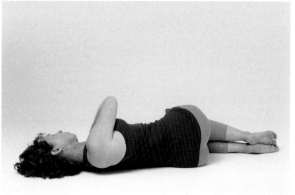

3. Then draw the right shoulder blade backwards towards the floor and allow a relaxed right arm to follow. Keep going until the whole of the right shoulder is flat on the floor. Let your shoulder blade, rib cage and pelvis follow as much as they need to allow the right shoulder to reach the floor comfortably. Then, if you have room, unfold the right arm so that it forms a straight line with the left arm.
4. Rewind the process to get back to your starting place, and repeat several times. Then swap sides.

SENSE OF ENQUIRY
- As you go through the movement, does your head stay resting as it rolls on the floor?
- Do your lower ribs stay on the floor throughout the movement?
- Can you stay completely relaxed throughout the movement?

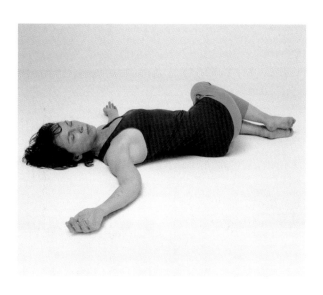

HAPPY BABY TURNING

PURPOSE
- To improve the mapping of rotation throughout the body.
- To improve the compliance of the body in turning.

APPROACHING THE ASANA
1. Lie on your back and take hold of your big toes between your legs (note: it is only worth doing this movement if you can reach your toes comfortably with your head on the floor).
2. Turn your head to the right and invite the body to follow until you are completely on your right side.
3. Then turn your head round to the left and invite your body to follow the movement until you are completely on your left side.
4. Go from side to side as smoothly and comfortably as possible.

SENSE OF ENQUIRY
- Do you lift either the head or lower ribs off the floor as you go through the movement?
- Is the movement smooth and flowing?
- Does your breathing remain comfortable and easy?

'Turn your head to the right and invite the body to follow…
Go from side to side as smoothly and comfortably as possible.'

KNEELING TURN

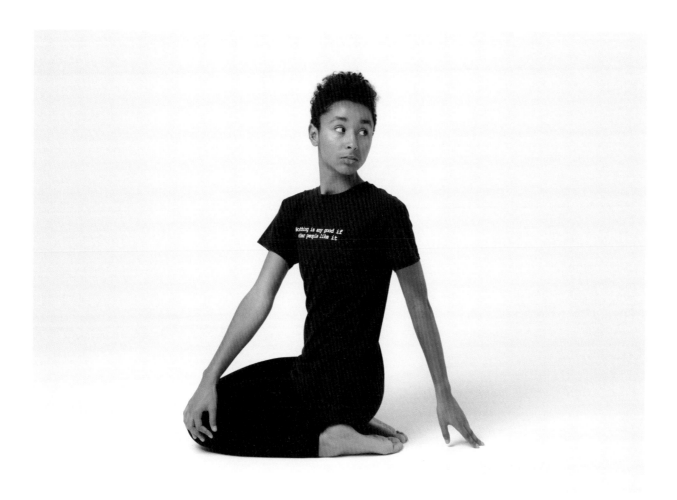

PURPOSE
- To help map the movement of the shoulder girdle, rib cage and spine in turning.

APPROACHING THE ASANA
1. Sit on your heels and make yourself comfortable. You might want to use a blanket for support under your ankles or between your heels and sitting bones.
2. Rock the pelvis a little backwards (flexion) and then a little forwards (extension), finally coming to a place where you feel you are doing neither.
3. Turn your head to the left and allow the shoulders and rib cage to follow.
4. If it is comfortable, place your right hand towards the outside of the left knee, and support yourself with the left hand on the floor a little behind you.
5. Repeat on the other side.

SENSE OF ENQUIRY
- As you turn your head to the left, notice how the movement travels through your spine down to the pelvis.
- Notice how the left and right shoulder blades move as you turn to the left, and allow the arms to follow the shoulder blades rather than lead them.
- Once the turn has reached its comfortable limit, bring the hands into the position described.
- Notice how the turn develops a little as you exhale, and how it reduces a little as you inhale.

WIDE-STRIDE TURN

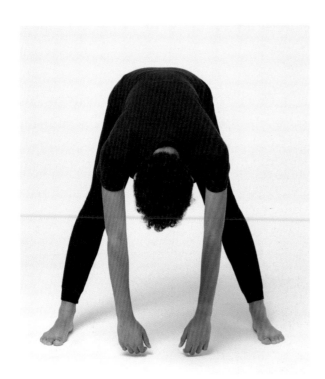

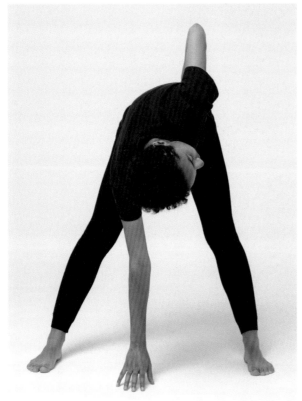

PURPOSE
- To help map the movement of turning in the spine, shoulders and rib cage.

APPROACHING THE ASANA
1. Stand with the legs comfortably wide apart, and bend forwards so the trunk is parallel with the floor. Keep the legs straight unless your hamstrings are too tight, in which case allow the knees to bend.
2. Fold a little further and bring the hands to the floor in front of you. Turn your head to the left and allow the body to follow. Bring the right hand to the floor below your shoulder.
3. When you have turned as far as is comfortably possible, reach up with the left arm but be careful not to use it to lever yourself further round. If it feels a strain to bring the left arm up, rest it on the sacrum instead (as shown in the photo).
4. Repeat the movement several times, and then do the same movement to the right.

SENSE OF ENQUIRY
- Do not allow strain to build up in the shoulders when you reach up with the arms.
- Notice whether you are turning or turning and looking back when you start the movement.

'When you have turned
as far as is comfortably possible,
reach up with the left arm but
be careful not to use it to lever
yourself further round.'

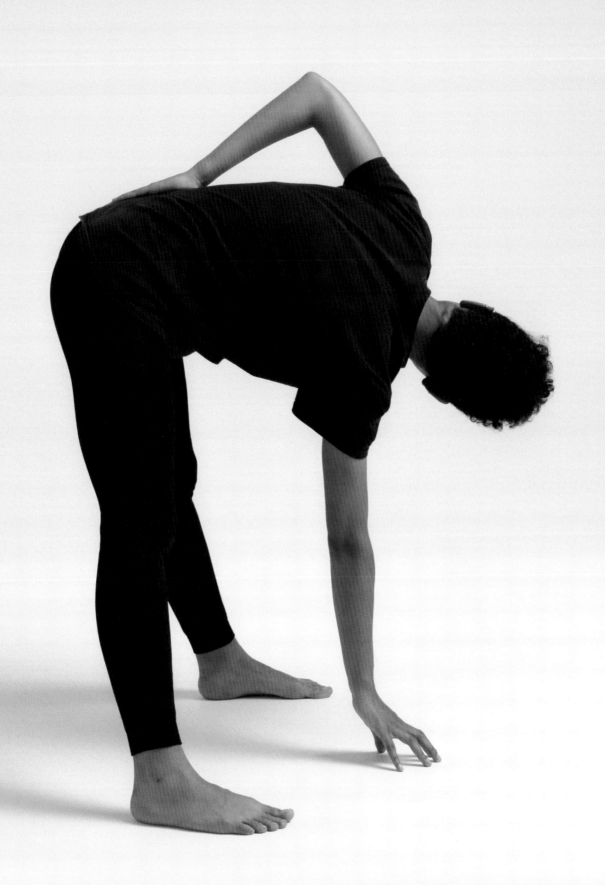

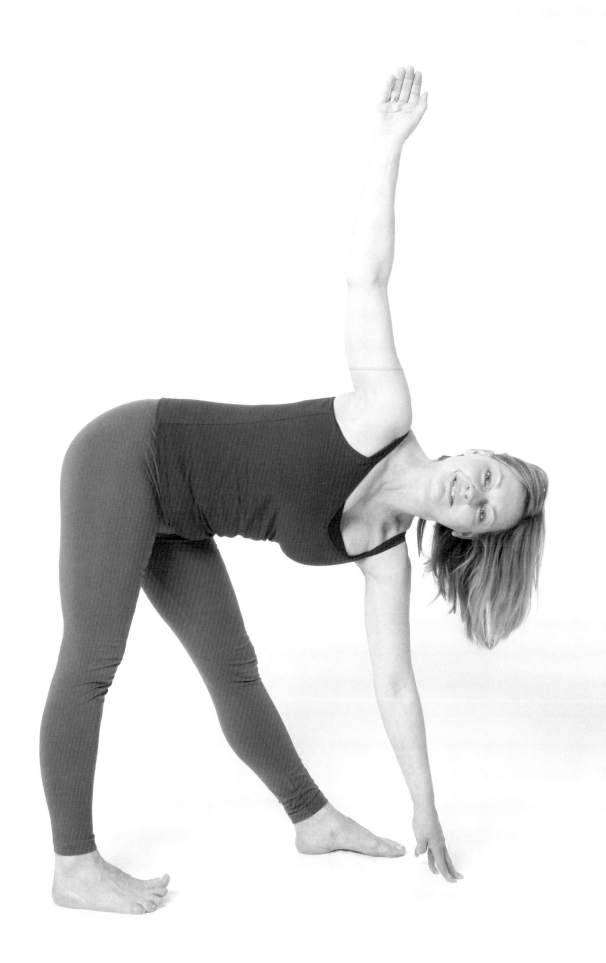

BENDING-FORWARD TWIST

These movements add a bit more complexity to turning movements. The premise of any movement needs to be stability and the ability to quieten the nervous system before doing anything else. Here we are trying to maintain the stability we find in Sprinter (p.115) and maintain it while we turn the body. It is often when we move the head that we lose stability and start to wobble, so the practice here is to maintain that stability while introducing the turn.

What to do with the pelvis as you turn? There is no particular rule here, but it is helpful to recognise the two main possibilities: you can keep the pelvis still (constraint) to direct the turning movement into the spine; or you can allow the pelvis to follow the turn (compliance), where the turn is shared between the pelvis and spine. It may be that some people will benefit from focusing the movement in their spine, while others would need to distribute movements more evenly.

PURPOSE
To help map our stability while developing compliance in turning.

APPROACHING THE ASANA
This movement can be approached in a variety of ways. In the past, I have viewed it as separate movements, but I am now more inclined to think of the asana as two related postures that you can move in and out of as feels appropriate. There are two main ways to come into this movement: from Sprinter pose or from standing.

STARTING IN SPRINTER
1. In Sprinter pose (p.115), rest the pelvis back onto the left foot and find stability through the right foot. Map the whole footprint and relax your body as best you can.
2. Slowly straighten your left leg and settle the foot

onto the floor, again taking time to find the footprint on the floor.
3. Bring the right hand to the floor somewhere near the front right foot and turn your head as though to look up the wall to your left. Keeping your feet stable, let the body follow the movement of the head until you are looking more towards the ceiling.
4. Then, if it is comfortable, reach up with your left arm but try not to use it as a lever to increase your sense of 'turn'.

STARTING FROM STANDING
5. Take your right foot forwards one comfortable step, and settle into your footprints until you feel stable.
6. Bend forward and bring your hands to the floor on either side of your foot.
7. Follow points three and four above.

SENSE OF ENQUIRY
- Are you able to keep yourself quiet and steady as you turn your body?
- When you turn, do you notice if you also bend forwards?
- Is your breathing easy and relaxed throughout the movement?

Note: It does not matter too much whether you have the front leg straight or bent. Of course, if your hamstrings are very tight, straight legs might not be an option so the front leg would remain bent. If you do have the option and want to change from one to the other, keep some of your attention on your footprints as you move from bent to straight legs and vice versa. Of course, we can also turn the other way and turn towards the leading leg. This is a more difficult movement when the front leg is bent, and tends to ask more of the spine than the pelvis.

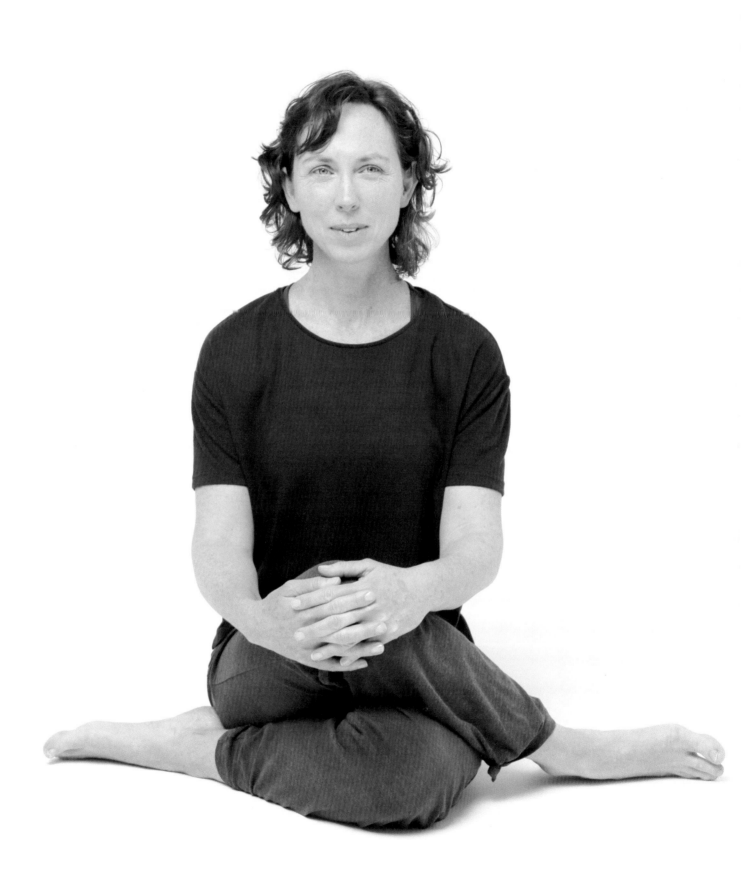

FUNCTIONAL ASANAS: SITTING

Sitting postures are important because they demand of the person doing them certain abilities that are disappearing from our modern culture. Chief amongst these is the ability to get up and down from the floor with ease. To be able to do this we need reasonably mobile feet and ankles, we need knees and hips that can flex and, perhaps most significantly, we need the strength in our legs to allow us to lift and lower our body weight. Getting down to sit on the floor, staying there for a bit and then getting up again involves a straightforward set of movements that we should strive to maintain for as long as possible. A Brazilian study undertaken in 2012 by Dr Claudio Gil Araújo and colleagues at the Clinimex Exercise Medicine Clinic in Rio de Janeiro showed that people who maintained this ability had a significantly better health prognosis than those who had lost the ability. If you can do this movement, then another repertoire of activities remains available to you – meaning that you are able to remain active for longer. And being active is, as we know, one of the strongest correlates to a healthy life. So, if nothing else, practise improving the way you come up and down from the floor, paying attention until you have worked out the most comfortable way.

Over the years I have become less of a fan of sitting postures done with straight legs, as I explain on page 107. This is because so many people do not have sufficient length in their hamstrings to do these postures without creating a lot of tension in their hip flexors and lower back – and sitting with that kind of tension is simply not helpful. So I am focusing more on the sitting positions that require the knees and hips to be more involved; this is also the way most people naturally sit on the floor.

If possible, try to find at least three ways of sitting that you feel reasonably comfortable in, so that you can move from one to the other when you start to feel a bit uncomfortable. However, as adults it can take a long time for the soft tissues to change sufficiently to make floor-sitting comfortable – and if we try to force it in any way, it will be our knees that suffer. Sitting takes patience and persistence and it is often a better strategy to sit for a short while one way, and then to move and sit in a different way.

IN THIS SECTION

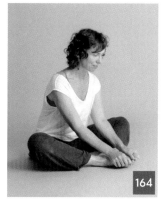

164

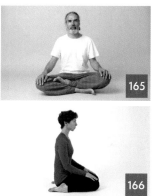

165

166

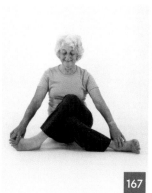

167

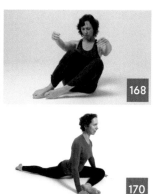

168

170

COBBLER POSE

Baddha Konasana

All sitting poses challenge the hips and knees in some way, and Cobbler particularly emphasises abduction of the hip. This causes most people to round out in the lower back through the attachment of the pubofemoral ligaments and the long adductors of the thigh. So this asana is generally better done sitting against a wall. If you try to do this without back support, you have to engage the hip flexors – namely the illiopsoas – to sit reasonably straight; and because of their insertion into the lesser trochanter of the femur, it is impossible to relax the hips while you are sitting, a prerequisite for any freeing up of the hips to improve sitting.

PURPOSE

To help free the hips in abduction and external rotation, and thus help prepare them for sitting.

APPROACHING THE ASANA

1. Start by sitting with your back to a wall. Take the base of your spine as close to the wall as possible and bring the soles of the feet together. If you are reasonably free in the hips, have the heels a few inches away from the pubic bone. If your hips seem quite stiff, on the other hand, allow the feet to move further away from the pubic bone until you feel comfortable.
2. Allow the knees to relax down. If there is discomfort, some support under the knees is helpful. Over time – sometimes years – the knees will go lower and progress can be developed by starting to lean forward. But this is only worthwhile pursuing if the knees are nearly on the floor. Stay in the posture for as long as feels comfortable.

SENSE OF ENQUIRY

- Be sure to slowly let go of the muscles in the groin. If you find this difficult, rest back against the wall more.
- Allow the feet to open away from each other if they are inclined to do this.
- Does your back feel comfortable?
- Do you feel you have enough space around your abdomen or do you feel a little slumped? If it is the latter, sit yourself closer to the wall.

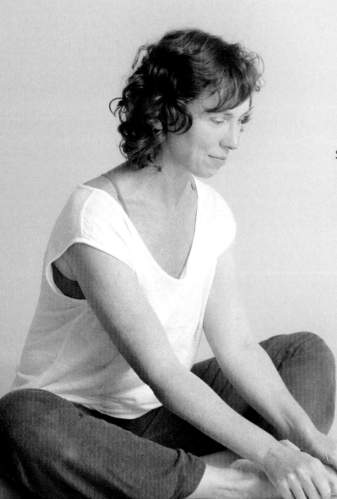

CROSS-LEGGED SITTING

Padmasana, Lotus or Half Lotus

———

The ease with which we sit cross-legged is to some extent related to the shape of the hip joint – which can have considerable individual variation – and also to the tension in the muscles and ligaments that surround the hip joint. However, it should be remembered that the musculo-ligamentous structures tend to modify themselves in line with use. So, if you sit cross-legged from an early age, those tissues will change accordingly. But if the bony configuration of the hip joint is not so well orientated for cross-legged sitting, chances are that as a child you would not instinctively choose this way to sit and so the soft tissues will then be less likely to accommodate this way of sitting as an adult.

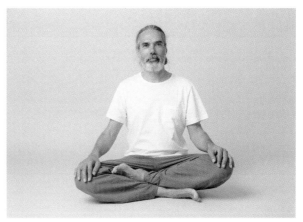

PURPOSE

Finding comfortable ways to sit on the floor requires persistence and practice, especially if we have not done it for a long time. Cross-legged sitting will be the preferred way for many people. It puts hips, knees and ankles through a useful range of movements that helps maintain their health.

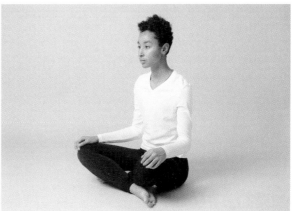

APPROACHING THE ASANA

1. Try to lean forwards with legs crossed. This can be a useful way to help release the hips for sitting. When we sit cross-legged, or in Lotus or Half Lotus, half the battle is getting your body weight forward of the gravity line. When we can do this, the hip flexors can relax, allowing greater freedom in the groin. (If we cannot bring our body past the vertical, we need the hip flexors to be active to keep us from slumping backwards – and when this happens our back will quickly tire.)

2. From the leaning forwards position, gradually walk the hands in and send the weight back into the sitting bones.

3. From here, sense that you are stacking your vertebra one over the other, sending the weight down through your spine into your sitting bones. In a very real sense you are sitting 'down' not 'sitting up'.

4. Find out how vertical you can become before you engage the muscles in the groin (illiopsoas), and stop just before that point. You want to be able to sit as tall as possible with the groin quiet.

SENSE OF ENQUIRY

- If you start to ache in the back, lean forwards onto your hands until the discomfort passes. Then, slowly stack your spine back up over the sitting bones.

- If you find you cannot lean forwards, sit with your back to the wall and rest against it.

- If your knee, foot or ankle starts to ache, it is best to change positions rather than try and sit it through.

- How upright do you feel? Look for the point where you feel most upright and with the least tension in your back.

———

SITTING BETWEEN THE HEELS
(HERO)
Virasana

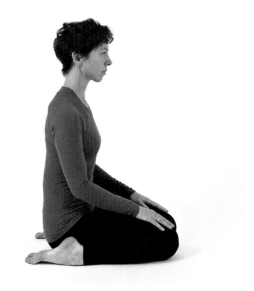

This sitting position tends to cause controversy in yoga circles because it is sometimes argued that it unavoidably puts strain on the structures of the knee. However, it is also true that many children tend to adopt this sitting position quite naturally without causing any apparent harm.

Much of the confusion is almost certainly due to the fact that the bony structure of the hip joint varies so much from individual to individual. In some people it facilitates internal rotation of the thigh, in others external rotation. To be able to sit comfortably between your feet, your hips need to be able to internally rotate fairly easily. To sit cross-legged they need to be able to externally rotate. So you often notice that people favour one or the other.

It is also worth remembering that although the knee is usually considered to be a hinge joint, its mechanics are far from a hinge action. It has components of both rotation and adduction/abduction, and when it goes through its main movement of flexion/extension, the femur glides on the tibia rather than hinges on it. If you think of the joint as a hinge, as many people do, sitting between your feet makes no sense because it would seem that you are putting strain on the hinge. If, however, our understanding is that the knee has aspects of multi-dimensional movement, this position seems less threatening and almost certainly helpful in maintaining the extension aspects of knee mechanics. I would like to emphasise, though, that the way an individual's hips are configured is the main influence on whether this asana feels comfortable or not.

PURPOSE

For those who find this asana reasonably comfortable, it maintains freedom of the inner knee – particularly the medial collateral ligaments. It also helps maintain plantar flexion at the ankle and flexion at the knee.

APPROACHING THE ASANA

1. Start by sitting on your heels and slide the feet apart so that they are beside the legs, close to the hips. If this feels uncomfortable on the knees, try placing a block or folded blanket under the sitting bones to take the weight of the body.
2. If there is discomfort at the knees when you start, you can take some weight through the arms to reduce the strain, and notice if the feeling eases. If so, relax the arms and bring them onto your lap.
3. The other thing that can affect the comfort of the knees is the orientation of the hips. Tucking the tail under a little may ease some discomfort at the knee. Conversely, if the pelvis is tipped forwards too much it may increase the feeling of strain. It is worth playing around with the position of the pelvis to find the most comfortable place for the knees whilst being as upright as possible.

SENSE OF ENQUIRY

- Does your spine feel reasonably upright without tension? Do your knees and feet feel comfortable? If there is some discomfort on the inside of the knee, it is worth putting a small lift under the sitting bones, until the knee discomfort goes.
- If the discomfort is more on the outside of the knee it can be worth trying putting a small folded cloth or belt tight into the back of the outside of the knee so you create a little more space there when you sit. If this takes the discomfort away use the folded cloth/belt for a few weeks and the discomfort should slowly subside.

LEGS CROSSED AT THE KNEES

Gomukasana

PURPOSE

This is perhaps the only seated posture that brings the spine and pelvis into an upright position without needing much muscular effort – and for that reason alone it is worth practising.

APPROACHING THE ASANA

There are two main ways into this asana: either start from sitting, with your legs in front of you and your knees bent and feet on the floor; or, it can be approached from all fours.

FROM SITTING

1. Start by sitting with your legs in front of you and your knees bent with your feet on the floor.
2. Rest back a little onto your hands, and bring your right knee over your left knee. Then, slide your left heel towards your right hip and then your right heel towards your left hip. Depending on how much freedom you have on the outside of the hip, you will find that as you gather the feet in towards your hips you might find your pelvis tipping to the side so that it becomes difficult to feel level.
3. Once both feet are tucked in as close to the hips as possible, try to ease your pelvis until your sitting bones are evenly balanced on the floor. In truth this very rarely happens! Most people will feel slightly more weight on one sitting bone than the other. If there is only a slight difference, this can be a great way to sit for the spine.
4. Stay for as long as feels comfortable. Then repeat the whole thing with the left leg over the right.
5. It is fine if you need to take some weight onto your hands initially, but you should not be taking all the weight in your arms!

FROM ALL FOURS

1. Come onto all fours, and bring your right knee across your left calf, so that it sits on the ground to the left of your left knee. Tuck the right knee as tight up towards the right knee as possible.
2. Widen the feet as far away from each other as

possible, then slowly take your weight back and bring the pelvis to the floor between your heels. If this feels awkward, putting a block or some support under the pelvis can be helpful.

3. If this posture comes easily, play around with the position of the pelvis, tipping it forwards and backwards slightly until you find the very easiest position for the spine. You want to feel upright and open without tension building in the groin.

SENSE OF ENQUIRY

- In this way of sitting there is often a little discomfort on the outside of the hip joints. This often eases after some moments. If, on the other hand, the discomfort increases, it is better to change sides fairly frequently.
- If you find the posture almost impossible, try sitting with the left leg straight out in front of you and then bring the right foot across the left thigh and draw the heel towards the left hip. This one-sided version is often more approachable if your hips are stiff in this movement. Then repeat on the other side.

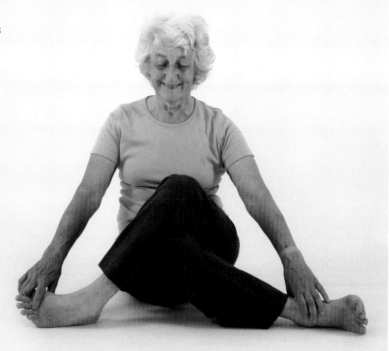

SIDE SITTING

This is one of the most useful ways of sitting, for several reasons. There is also a wide variety of ways to approach it. From a biomechanical point of view, it asks the hip joints to do different things. Whilst one hip joint needs to internally rotate, the other has to externally rotate. If you find that your pelvis is very uneven when on the ground, you have discovered that your internally rotating hip does not enjoy the movement and maybe your hips are more suited for external rotation movements. However, because the pelvis can easily lift if the hip is stiff, there is little danger to the knee when you do this, so it is a good way to encourage a decent range of hip rotation without endangering the knee.

The spine is also involved in this asana. Because it is asymmetrical, the spine will have a gentle 'C' curve in it when you sit one way, which will reverse when you put the legs to the other side. So it not only introduces a good range of movement to the hip joints, it also asks our spine to curve in both sideways directions. This is especially helpful as nearly all of us tend to have a dominant way we curve in our spines (our default scoliosis).

PURPOSE
To move the hip joints through both internal and external rotation, and to introduce side-bending in both directions to the spine. And, of course, to find a comfortable way of sitting.

APPROACHING THE ASANA
There are many ways to approach this, and each way brings something slightly different but useful to the asana.

FIRST METHOD (TOP IMAGES)
1. The most straightforward way is to start by sitting on your heels, then lean to your right, taking your weight onto the right hand.

2. Then, slide your feet from under your pelvis so they are nestled against the left hip. The left sitting bone will be off the ground and, to keep yourself in balance, you will have to lean a bit to the left, bringing a curve into your spine.
3. Then repeat this on the other side.
4. If this feels comfortable you can try doing it without leaning on your hands, using just the muscles of the legs and trunk.

SECOND METHOD (BOTTOM IMAGES)
1. Another, more complex way of coming into this sitting posture is to start by sitting with the legs in front of you, knees bent and feet on the floor.
2. Then lean back a little and support yourself with your hands behind you.
3. Swing your feet around to the left until they are as close to the left hip as possible, and sit yourself up as straight as possible.
4. Then, lean back on your hands and swing the feet all the way round to the right until they are as close to the right hip as possible.
5. If this feels fairly straightforward, try doing the same movement but without supporting yourself on your hands. This asks for a more complex mapping of the movement of the trunk muscles.

SENSE OF ENQUIRY
- If you approach this from sitting on your heels, make sure the knees feel comfortable. If there is any discomfort in the lower back, do not stay too long; rather, move from side to side without staying more than a moment in the sitting position.
- When you approach this with the legs in front of you, see how smoothly you can move the legs from one side to the other. Try not to let the feet brush against the floor as you swing them from hip to hip.

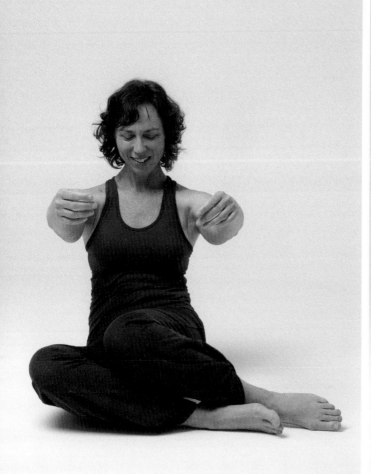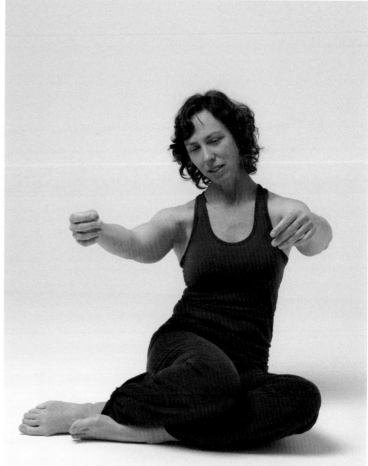
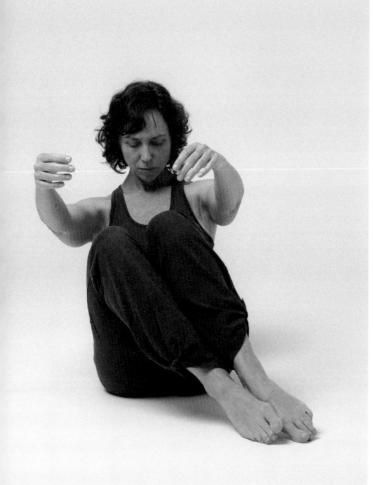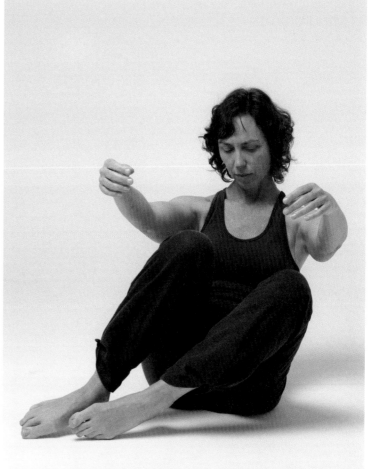

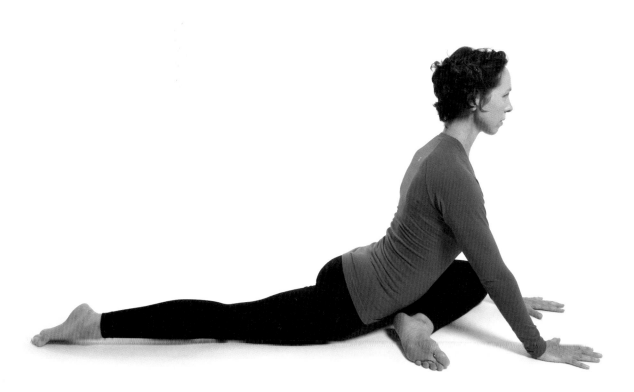

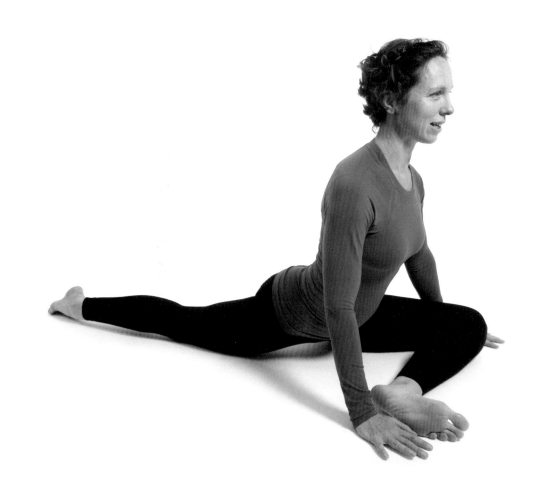

PIGEON

This is another posture that has its advocates and detractors. The criticism is usually concerned with the effect on the sacroiliac joint. Whilst there might be some justification for this in the hypermobile practitioner, the problems seem to develop if people stay for too long in the initial stage of the posture, or strive too hard in the extension part of the posture. For many people this can be a very helpful asana to help with sitting postures (in the first part of the pose), and extension movements (in the second part).

PURPOSE

There are two elements to this asana. In the initial part, the emphasis is on the hip and knee of the front leg, which is in a similar position to that needed for cross-legged sitting. The second part of the asana develops into an extension movement. By virtue of the fact that the front leg constrains the movement of the pelvis and therefore the lumbar spine in extension, it becomes easier to focus one's attention on the upper back without compressing the lumbar spine. So the two principal purposes are: to help the hip joint with external rotation, which is necessary for cross-legged sitting; and to map the extension movement in the upper thoracic spine.

APPROACHING THE ASANA

1. Come onto all fours and draw the right knee forwards as far as you comfortably can. Then, bring the right foot under the left thigh and take the right knee out to the right, so it is just a bit wider than the hip. Then slide the left leg back as far as possible, and rest your body over the right thigh. Do your best to keep the pelvis level.

2. Some people will find this gives a very strong feeling of stretch deep in the right buttock. If it is very uncomfortable, it is better to change sides fairly frequently rather than stay and suffer. If this part of the asana is comfortable, however, then it is worth walking the hands in until you are in a back bend – but not so far that there is any compression in the lumbar spine.

3. For a moment, check your support through the shoulders by sinking and then pushing through the shoulders, until you find a level of support that feels appropriate.

4. Then bring your gaze down to look at the floor. Notice how the pelvis subtly lifts a little at this point, then smoothly bring the gaze from the downward-looking position forwards and upwards until the gaze is just above the horizon line. As you do this, notice the pelvis moving a little towards the floor. Repeat the movement of looking down and then up in slow smooth movements, noticing the response of the pelvis to the movement of the head.

5. Repeat on the other side.

SENSE OF ENQUIRY

- Notice that the pelvis stays reasonably level from the floor as you go through the movements. Some people prefer to have the front foot dorsiflexed, others find it helpful to point the foot more. This will depend to some extent on the orientation of the hip joint and the state of your knee. What you are looking for is a position of the foot that makes the knee and hip feel most comfortable with a level pelvis.

- When taking the gaze down and up, does the rest of the body, and particularly the pelvis, join in easily?

'Bring your gaze down
to look at the floor. Notice how
the pelvis subtly lifts a little
at this point.'

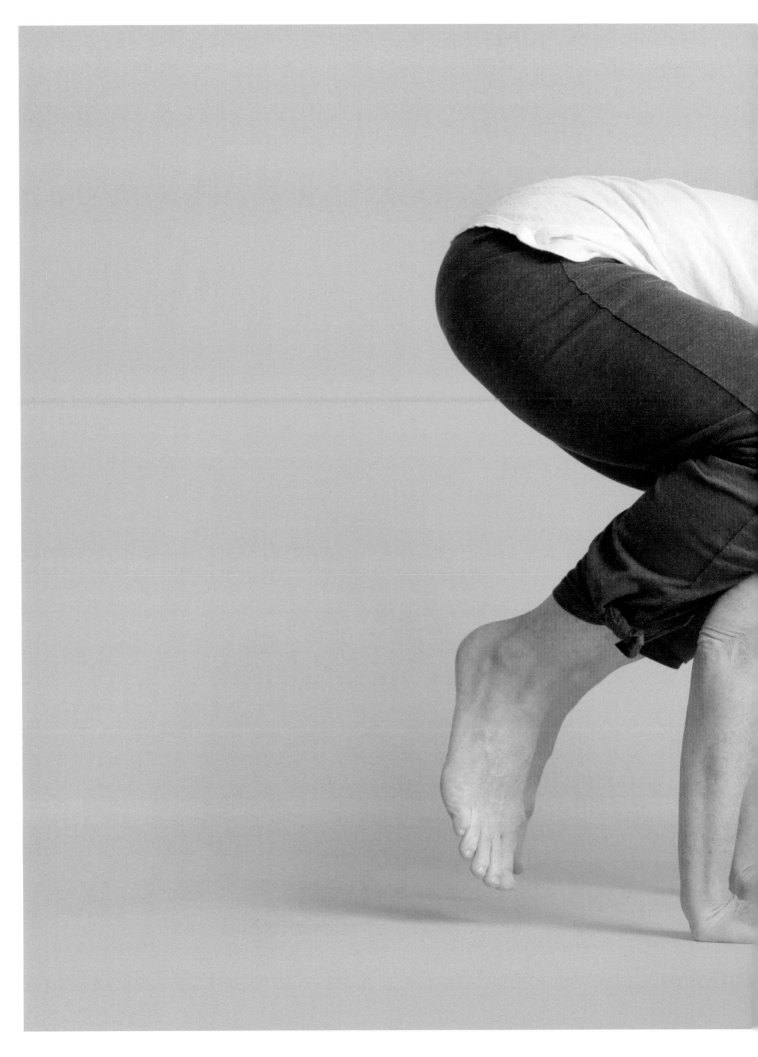

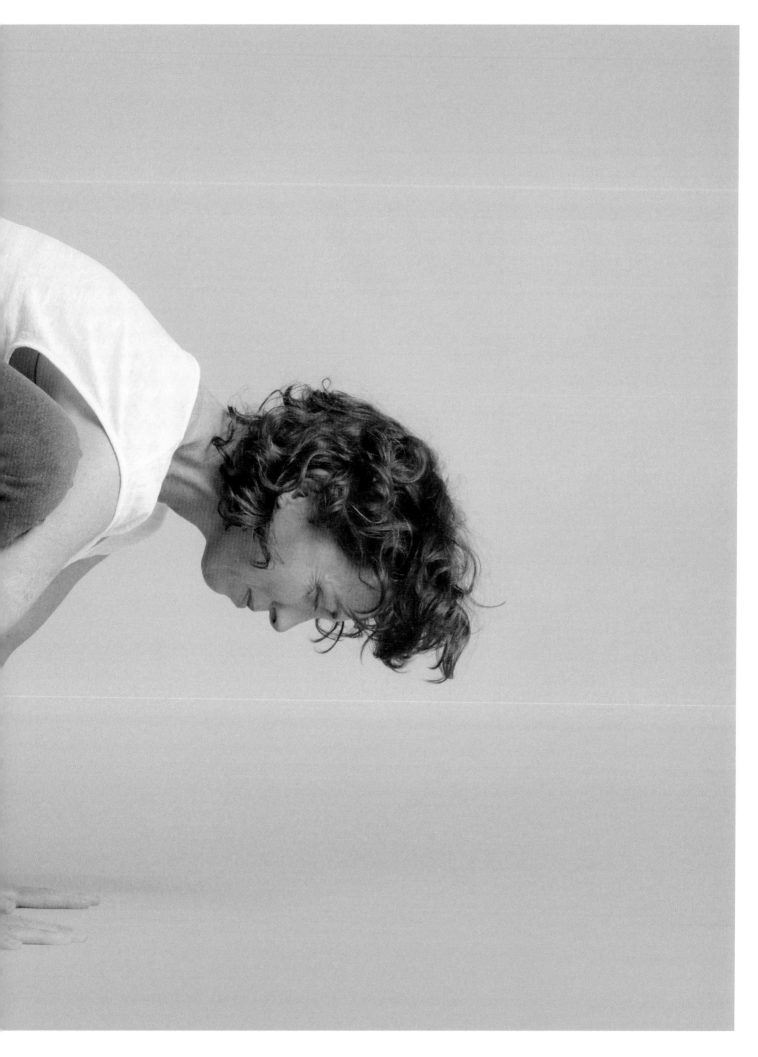

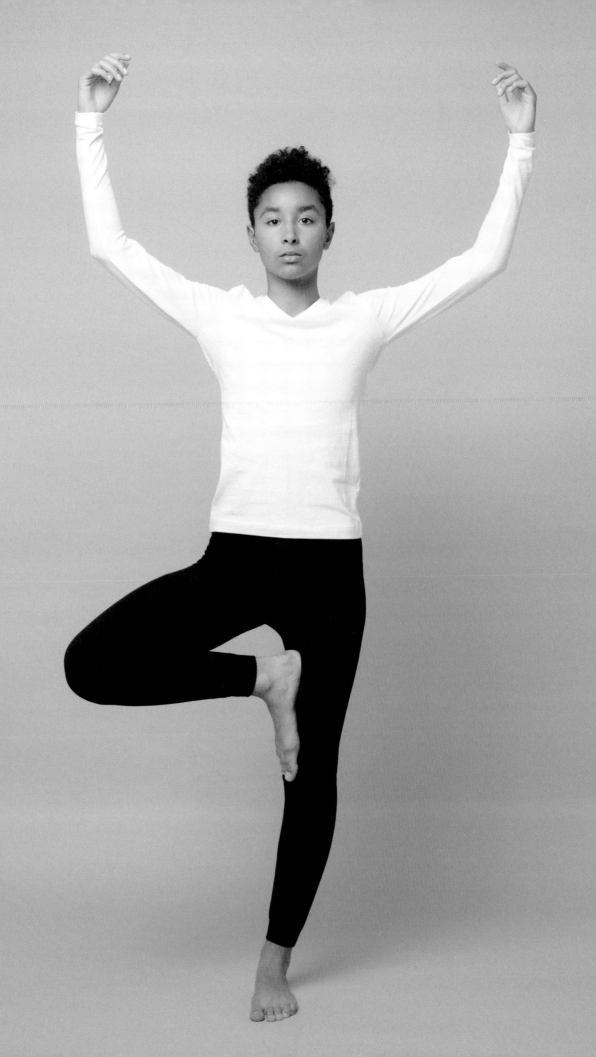

NINE

BALANCES

In recent years, health professionals have been asked to pay more attention to balance in the ageing population; it is becoming clearer that complications that develop from fractures after a fall put a significant burden on the healthcare system. While exercise and bone-loading movements are still seen as very important, improving balance is now considered to be of equal importance in improving long-term quality of life.

Balances are particularly useful in helping us understand grounding: so, how we meet the floor and how steady we become. In standing balances, the feet need to be strong and stable, the upper body free and responsive.

We tend to become tense and stiff when we feel unstable, and this is unhelpful – rigid structures topple more easily than responsive ones. The principal concern in balances is to develop poses slowly, steadily and with quiet stability.

Where possible, try to imagine weight being transmitted through the bones. These are the structures in the body that transmit forces. When we 'find' our bones, muscles can relax and movement becomes smoother and more effortless.

Balance also tends to get worse as we age, but it has been shown that regular practice can improve it a great deal. Thus the following asanas are well worth persevering with.

IN THIS SECTION

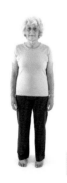
176

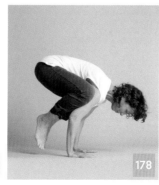
178

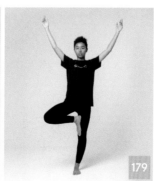
179

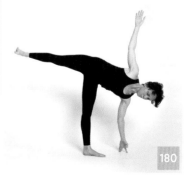
180

BALANCED STANDING POSE
(MOUNTAIN)

Tadasana

Learning to stand more comfortably is not always easy and has more to do with finding out how you are standing than with *trying* to stand up straight or 'correctly'. We write our lives into our bodies and the ways we hold ourselves, and the little tensions and holding patterns we have developed over a lifetime become unnoticed. So it makes no sense to say anybody stands 'badly', or to tell someone to stop doing whatever it is they are doing. What is more useful is to help people become familiar with the things they do. Only then is it really possible to address these patterns.

The following advice on approaching Mountain pose does not have to be done every time, but it is helpful to try it at least once a week.

PURPOSE

Learning to stand comfortably is a great asset. Many of us spend a good deal of time on our feet, yet feel quite uncomfortable if we have to stand still for any period of time. If we learn to stand with ease, we can take that into any action that arises out of standing.

APPROACHING THE ASANA

1. Stand with the feet about hip-width apart and roughly parallel. Notice the way the weight falls through your feet. Are you more on the outside or the inside of the footprint?
2. Allow your weight to fall more into the inner footprint so you become a bit flatfooted. Notice how that travels into the legs, pelvis and upper body. Let the feeling 'land'.
3. Then roll the weight to the outside of the feet so the footprint is mainly on the outer edge. Really *feel* the weight shift through your feet, and again follow the consequences through your legs, pelvis and upper body.
4. Finally, settle on the feeling of having your weight fairly even on the inner and outer footprint. Bring your attention to your knees, particularly the

kneecaps, and try lifting the kneecaps and then relaxing them. Do it several times until you feel you can stand with the knees relaxed. Be careful not to find the relaxed position by pushing through the knees and hyperextending. If you are a natural hyper-extender, think more about resting the thighbone above the shinbone.

5. Relax your arms and shoulders, then slowly relax your chin down as though you wanted to look at your navel. Let the breastbone sink and the shoulder blades slide forwards. Feel the hips swing back. Be in a really good slump. Feel it through your whole body, then slowly bring your gaze up from your navel towards the horizon. Notice how the spine starts to straighten, the breastbone starts to rise, the shoulders start to slide back and the pelvis starts to move back.
6. Then slowly start to bring the gaze to above the horizon, somewhere between the horizontal and right above you. Again notice your spine follow the head and neck into extension, feel the breastbone rise and the shoulders slide back and down a little. The pelvis will tend to swing forward. Allow it to.
7. Move slowly and smoothly between your gentle slump and looking up, sensing the movements of the breastbone, shoulder blades and pelvis.
8. Finally, settle on the place where, to the best of your ability, you sense you are neither slumping nor looking up. You want to get to the position where you are trying not to *do* something.

SENSE OF ENQUIRY

- Notice whether you feel discomfort, and if you do, try the gentle slump and extension movement a few times to see if you can ease it. If you are quite uncomfortable standing, only remain there briefly; do something else and come back to it.
- From time to time, bring your attention back to your footprints and see if the whole of each footprint is still represented on the ground.

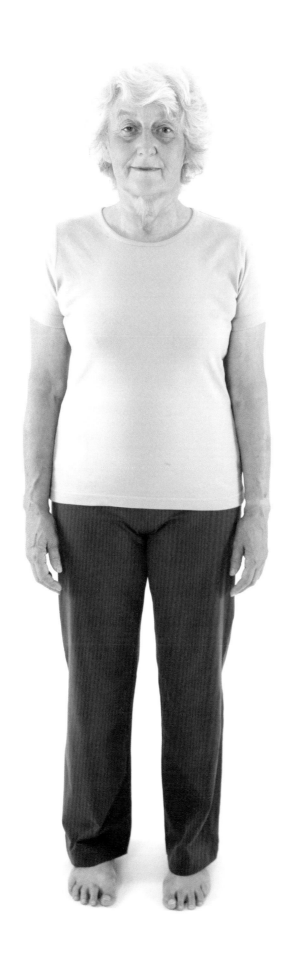

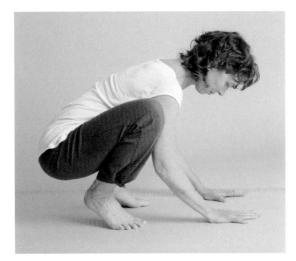

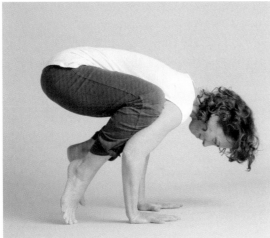

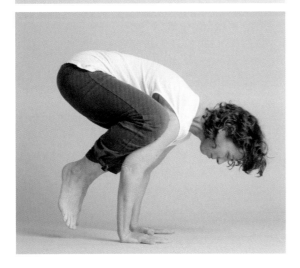

CROW POSE

Bakasana

This asana is not for everyone, and those with stiff or arthritic wrists might want to avoid it. But it is an interesting balance if your wrists will allow it.

PURPOSE

- To bring our attention to where our centre of gravity is, as we shift our weight onto our hands.
- To help distinguish tension from effort in more complex circumstances.

APPROACHING THE ASANA

1. Come onto your haunches and place your hands on the floor between your knees. Really find your handprints.
2. Come up onto your tip toes bringing your knees as high up the upper arms as possible, then rock gentle forwards and backwards from your toes. Notice how your wrists feel.
3. If your wrists feel okay, slightly grip your upper arm with your knees as you take your weight forwards onto your hands, until your feet feel light on the floor. Then draw the feet up under you.
4. You have two options for your gaze: looking down and through your legs, with the body tending to go into flexion as you take the weight onto your hands, or on the horizon as you bring the weight onto your hands. The latter tends to encourage a feeling of extension in the body, although it is unlikely to actually become a back bend. Try practising both ways to find a place where you feel most comfortable.

SENSE OF ENQUIRY

- Are you are bringing any more effort than is required for the action?
- When you bring your feet up under your body, think more from the knees than the hips.

ONE FOOT STANDING BALANCE
(TREE)
Vrksasana

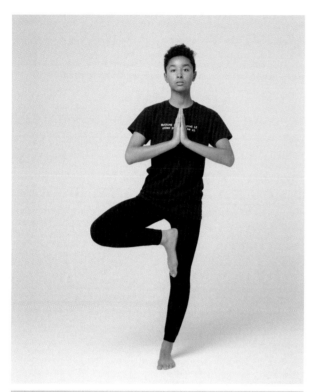

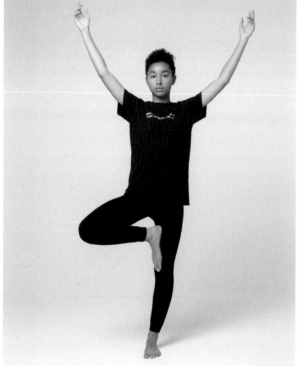

PURPOSE

To improve our sense of balance. As we age it is noticeable that in the population at large balance seems to get worse and many people sustain injuries through falls. In the very elderly this can be the start of a slippery slope: someone falls, injures themselves and, in the intervening weeks during the recovery, loses strength and mobility, rather quickly finding themselves feeling considerably worse off than before the fall. Balance really does improve with practice so it is worth persevering.

APPROACHING THE ASANA

1. Stand in Mountain and pay attention to the quiet, steady feeling in the feet. Try to develop it.
2. Slowly shift your weight onto your left foot, taking less weight on the right foot. If you continue to feel steady, bring the right foot off the ground and either place it on your left ankle or, if the hip and knee allows, bring the foot to rest on the inside of the left thigh. Nestle the foot into a comfortable place and allow the knee to drop towards the floor.
3. If you find balancing difficult, have the arms wide to help with the balance. As you become more stable you can raise the arms above your head and if this still feels okay, try bringing the hands into prayer in front of you. Stay there for at least 30 seconds if you can. If you become competent at this, try closing your eyes and seeing if you can maintain your balance for at least ten seconds.

SENSE OF ENQUIRY

- Remember, we are practising how to be steady on one leg, so if you are wobbling in your balance, come down and steady yourself again so you feel quiet again. Do not simply practise wobbling!
- Does your standing foot feel quiet and stable throughout the movement?
- Do you feel reasonably even from the inner to outer footprint throughout the movement?

SIDEWAYS STANDING BALANCE
(HALF MOON)

Ardha Chandrasana

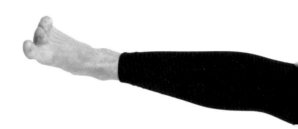

PURPOSE

- To develop one's sense of balance and stability, whilst doing slightly more challenging things with your body.
- To help differentiate the pelvis from the femur.

APPROACHING THE ASANA

1. Start in Mountain (p.176), and then reach your hands to the floor a little in front of your feet; bend your knees if you need to.

2. Find your footprints, and gradually shift your weight onto the left foot. Keep it quiet and steady on the floor.

3. Raise the right leg up behind you keeping the leg fairly straight but not obsessively so. Keep the weight through the standing leg with a quiet steady foot. Use the hands as stabilisers rather than to lean on.

4. Whilst keeping your hands on the floor, try lifting your right hip above your left hip and then bring it back to the starting position again. Lift and lower the right hip slowly and smoothly several times while you keep the standing foot quiet and steady.

5. Once this feels okay and you can lift and lower the pelvis easily without disturbing your standing foot, take the right hand off the floor and slide it slowly along the left arm and the top of your chest, and then reach the arm up without pulling it back. Let the trunk turn with the arm until you are facing the wall in front of you with your body.

6. Stay here briefly before returning the hand to the floor and turning the trunk and pelvis back to face the floor. Keep your gaze looking at the floor throughout the movement.

7. Repeat this several times until you feel you can turn the trunk and return it with the standing foot remaining stable.

'See if you can make the movement of the hip lifting and lowering smooth and fluid.'

8. Finally, add turning the head, either with the movement of the trunk or after the movement of the trunk. When turning the head, do your very best, again, to keep the footprint stable. Then repeat on the other side.

SENSE OF ENQUIRY

- Notice at what point in the movement you start to feel wobbly – it is that moment that you should practise until you feel stable again.
- Notice if you inadvertently shift the weight onto your hands as you go through the movement. Try to keep the weight through your standing footprint.
- See if you can make the movement of the hip lifting and lowering smooth and fluid.

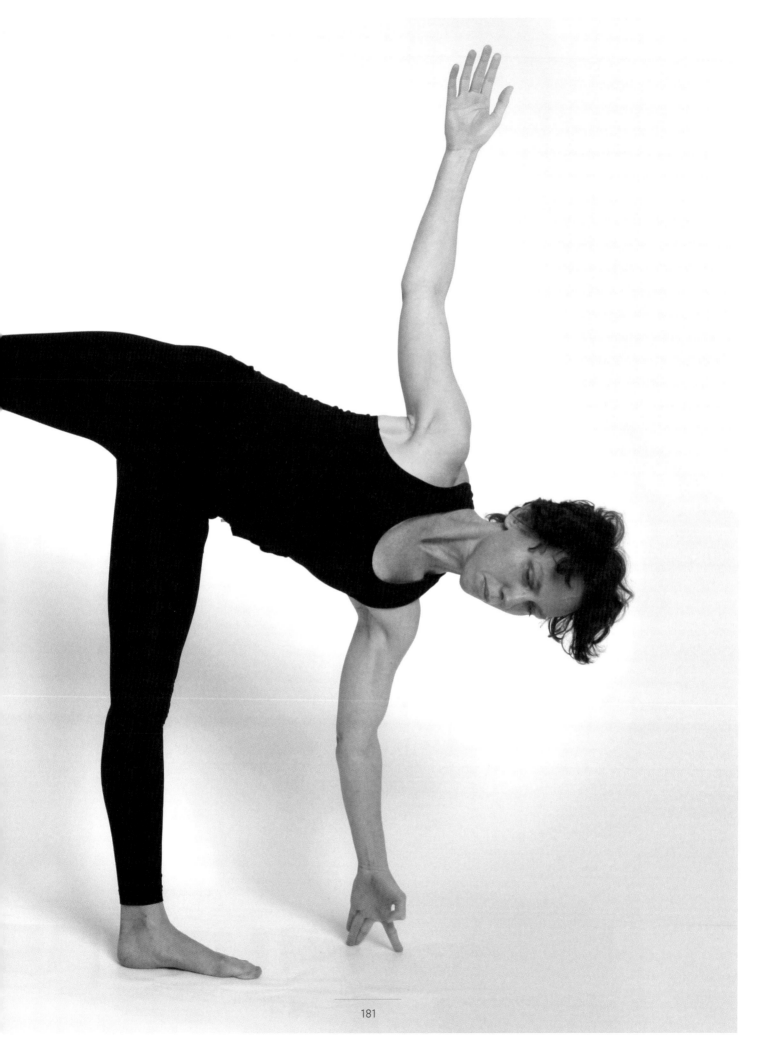

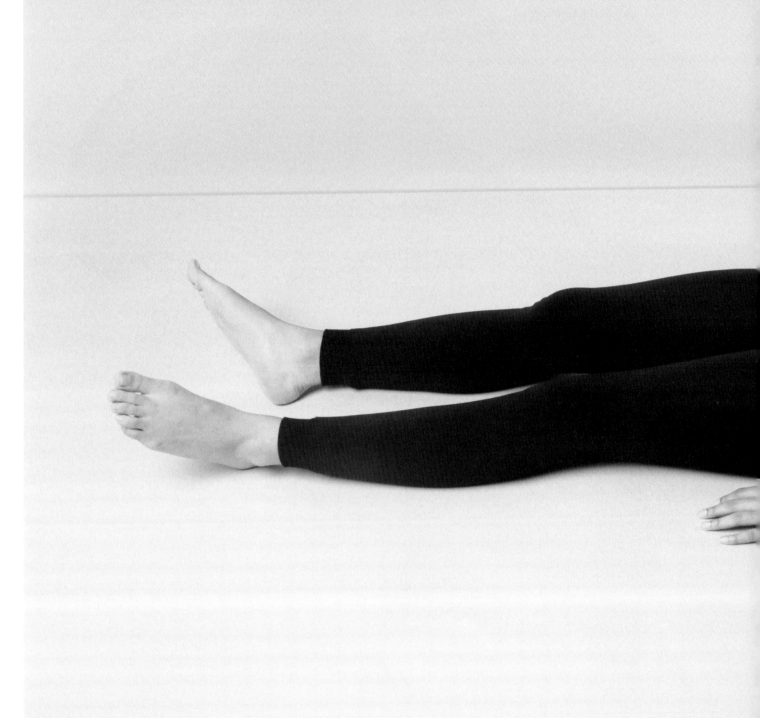

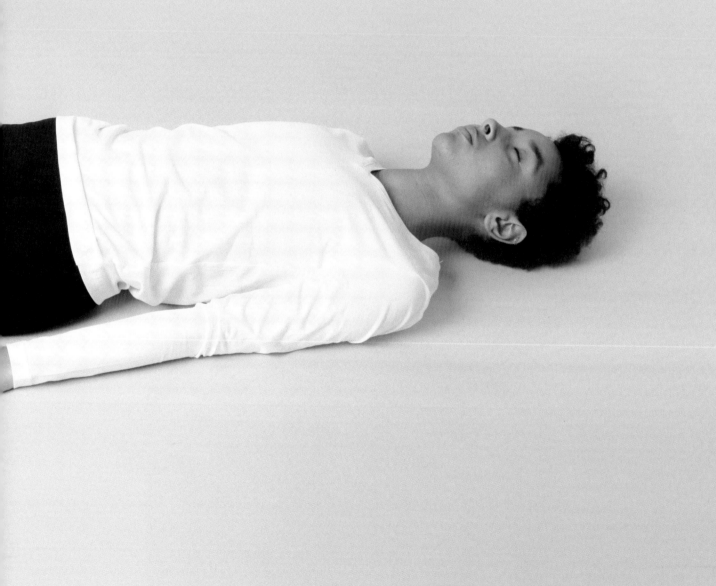

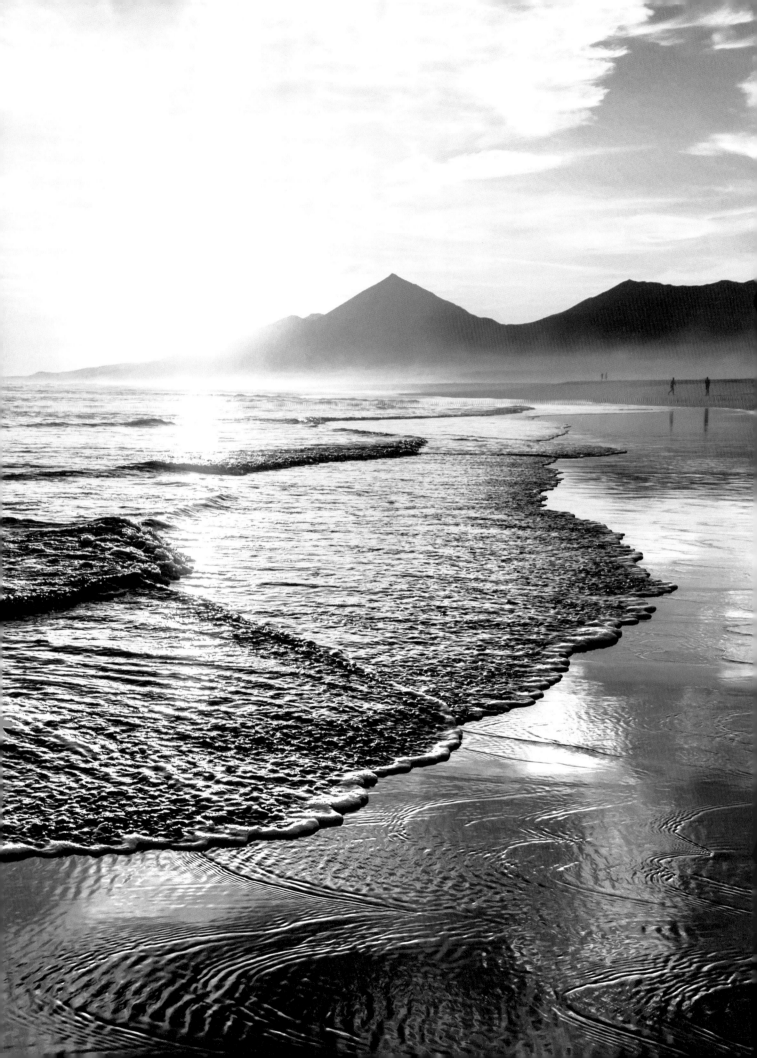

───── TEN ─────

RE-FINDING OUR BREATH
Breathing techniques and relaxation

Many techniques developed in yoga are designed to bring equilibrium back to the respiratory system. While the asanas can help re-map the muscles supporting respiration, some muscles are more difficult to notice than others. These include the diaphragm, the pelvic floor and the transverse abdominus – the respiratory muscles that support the fluid core of the body. It is here, therefore, that a more specialised approach is required, namely a mixture of breathing practices and bandha work (control of the respiratory muscles), together with some *kriyas* (cleansing techniques). The two techniques that I think are most helpful for this are Uddiyana bhanda and Kapalabhati.

As I explained in chapter three, it is important to recognise the relationship between breathing and movement. When we lie on our backs with our knees bent and feet on the floor, the whole body is supported by the ground, so we need no muscular response to gravity. The body will choose the easiest way to breathe, meaning that breathing here will always move into the softest part of the trunk. This is nearly always the abdomen. Abdominal ('diaphragmatic') breathing only requires activity in the diaphragm; the abdominal muscles have to relax.

If we breathe into the chest in this semi-supine position, we move away from the natural response to a conscious one. This can be a useful enquiry, as we soon find out if there is any resistance to breathing. While most people will find abdominal breathing easier in this position, chest breathing should not

feel difficult. If we alternate between taking a 'belly breath' and a 'chest breath' a few times, we soon get a sense of the type of breathing we have habituated. For 'chest breathers', it can be useful to lie with one hand on the belly and the other on the ribs, and to practise quiet breathing, allowing only the belly to move. If you cannot breathe into the chest without the belly moving, it can be helpful to practise chest breathing with the arms over the head. When we do this, the muscles running from the arms and shoulders to the ribs and lower back help to elevate the ribs mechanically. This encourages the breath to move more into the thorax and less into the belly.

It is interesting to note that when we come on to all fours, there is a natural tendency to tighten the abdominal muscles and in so doing unconsciously prevent the spine from collapsing. Again, this is a reflex change, the body's response to gravity, which again impacts on breathing. These reflex changes are a sign of well-integrated breathing and will tend to occur when unnecessary effort is reduced to a minimum.

To lose unnecessary tension we need to find adequate support from our bones; we need to become well-grounded. When we are well-grounded, but not stiff, we may be still but the slightest impulse could initiate movement. Conversely, any unhelpful muscle tension will stiffen us and take the potential for movement away. In well-grounded movements, breathing can adjust appropriately, whereas stiffness tends to 'fix' breathing.

UDDIYANA BHANDA

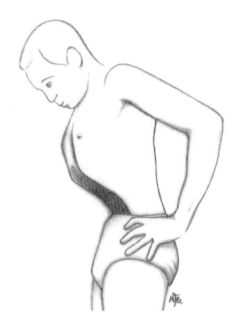

PURPOSE

This is the only way, as far as I'm aware, of consciously drawing the diaphragm up, something we can lose if we are anxious and holding on tightly with this muscle. Although Uddiyana bhanda is something children naturally experiment with, a lot of people lose the capacity to do it as they age.

We need to be prepared to experience the respiratory system doing unfamiliar things in this exercise, which should be taken slowly and thoughtfully.

To prepare the body for this posture, one needs to be able to experience the respiratory system doing unfamiliar things. The following breathing exercises are very useful for this. They should be taken slowly and thoughtfully.

APPROACHING THE TECHNIQUE

1. Lying on your back with the knees bent and the feet on the floor, breathe into the belly and keep the rib cage quiet and undisturbed. This contracts the diaphragm while relaxing the belly.
2. Breathe into the chest and keep the belly quiet. This activates the rib elevator muscles, with less activity in the diaphragm.
3. Alternate between the two exercises above: one breath into the belly, the next one into the chest.
4. Now try to make the belly-breath movement without breathing – expanding the belly while not actually breathing in. This is a voluntary contraction of the diaphragm with inhibition of the rib elevator muscles.
5. Try the same with the chest breath. Expand the rib cage but do not actually breathe in. This is a voluntary contraction of the rib elevator muscles that inhibits the activation of the diaphragm.
6. Exhale fully and pause the breath at the end of the exhalation. Note the tension that builds up in the abdominal muscles when you exhale fully, acknowledging how the abdominals act as accessory muscles for deep exhalation by pulling the ribs together.

7. Now see if you can exhale fully and relax the abdominal muscles while the breath is held at the end of the out-breath. To do Uddiyana Bandha successfully, the breath needs to be fully out, but the abdominals must be relaxed.
8. Now do all the steps to stage 7, and with the breath still paused, expand the rib cage as you did in stage 5. Your abdomen will feel drawn in, because the expanded rib cage will have lowered the pressure inside the thoracic cavity and the diaphragm will be drawn up into it. The abdominal organs, abdominal wall and the pelvic floor will all move up as well. You are now doing Uddiyana bhanda. It can be helpful to practise this with the arms on the floor above the head, as this helps elevate the ribs. Not only does Uddiyana bhanda stretch a tight diaphragm, it also draws up abdominal organs and takes pressure off the pelvic floor, both of which are compromised by a low diaphragm.

POINTS TO NOTE

There are some contraindications for Uddiyana bhanda, namely inflammatory conditions of the gut including diverticulitis, Crohn's disease and ulcerative colitis. Conditions such as irritable bowel syndrome (IBS) may improve with gentle Uddiyana work, as may many other digestive disorders. It is inadvisable to practise this during pregnancy, or if it causes discomfort during menstruation.

KAPALABHATI

PURPOSE

Kapalabhati can help us notice and re-map our relationship with the transverse abdominal muscles and the pelvic floor. This breathing exercise, or *kriya*, is described differently in different books. Here, I describe the technique where the exhalation is the active part of the breath and the inhalation is passive. It has some useful and beneficial effects, which I will explore here.

APPROACHING THE TECHNIQUE

1. Sit in a comfortable position and place your fingertips about halfway between your navel and your pubic bone.

2. Image you are going to blow out a candle flame with one short, sharp breath. Feel what your abdominal muscles do. They should move in. (A few people will find that the muscles move out instead, which is a very inefficient way of expelling air.) The main muscle that should contract here is the transverse abdominal. It squeezes in, forcing the contents of the abdomen to move up against the diaphragm, which in turn pushes on the lungs from below and forces air out of them. This movement activates the transverse abdominal muscle and relaxes the diaphragm, the opposite of what so often happens in daily life, where a tense diaphragm pushes down on weakened abdominal muscles.

3. Practise blowing out your imagined candle five to ten times with a second's pause between each one, each time with a sharp inward contraction of the abdomen. The in-breath comes in passively if you relax the abdomen between each exhalation. With practice, you should be able to blow out many times without running out of breath.

4. When you can do at least twenty exhalations comfortably, repeat the process but breathe out through the nose instead of the mouth. This is Kapalabhati.

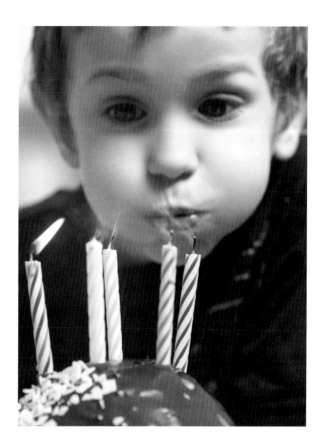

ABOVE
It can help to imagine that you are blowing out a candle flame with one short, sharp breath.

POINTS TO NOTE

If the idea of blowing out a candle does not work, you can try making a 'ha' sound, which will produce a similar response in the abdomen. Although not traditionally taught this way, I tend to encourage people, especially women, to practise Kapalabhati with concomitant contraction of the pelvic floor, i.e. bringing in an aspect of Mula bhanda into the exhalation. When the abdomen is drawn in during exhalation, the abdominal contents are pushed upwards, helping expel air from the lungs. However, like the toothpaste tube that is squeezed in the middle, some of the contents will also move down against the pelvic floor. This is unhelpful and may even exacerbate problems such as stress incontinence, prolapse or haemorrhoids. Do not keep the pelvic floor muscles lifted continually, rather contract and release them with the abdominal muscles. This will bring some tone to the pelvic floor as well as the abdominal muscles.

SUPINE RELAXATION

Savasana

PURPOSE

To allow the body to relax completely. The ability to lose tension in the muscles is an important part of yoga practice. As I have mentioned before, we can only relax a muscle if it is supported. In Savasana, we find as much support from the floor as possible to facilitate this and, significantly, really try to notice how it feels. It becomes the reference point for many other asanas; we notice tension and effort in reference to a relaxed body. Only if we know how it feels to be relaxed can we measure with any accuracy the amount of effort or tension we are holding.

APPROACHING SAVASANA

1. Lie on the floor with the legs a little apart and the arms by your side, comfortably away from the body. Ease the back of your head away from your shoulders, then let your neck relax, widen your shoulder blades away from each other, then release them. Ease the back of your pelvis towards your feet and then release the pelvis. Look for the support of the floor through the bony points of contact – namely, the back of the head, across the shoulders, the back of the pelvis and the points of contact on the floor through the arms and legs.

2. Turn the hands and arms so the palms face up and see how it feels. Then turn them so the palms face down, and see how it feels. Repeat several times quite quickly and then let the arms rest where they feel most comfortable.

3. Keeping the left heel on the floor, lift the left knee about five centimetres off the floor, and then let it drop back to the floor. Repeat with the right leg. Go from knee to knee, lifting and dropping them alternately with increasing speed, until you feel you are stamping your knees like a two-year-old having a tantrum. As soon as you feel your legs getting a bit tired drop both knees to the floor, unbend your legs and let go of them completely.

4. Then turn your legs so the toes point towards each other. And then turn them until the toes turn away from each other. Go from turning in to turning out rapidly until you are doing the movement almost as fast as you can. When your legs start to feel a bit tired, stop the movement and let go of the legs completely.

5. Wait a few moments and notice how you feel. If you need to make any adjustments to the body to become more comfortable, make them.

6. Once you feel the body has become quiet, bring your attention to the spaces in the body. Start with the head: imagine spaciousness inside the head, widthways from ear to ear, and then from the front to back of the skull. Then take your attention to the eyes. You can close them if that feels okay, or leave them open if closing them disturbs you. Either way, imagine you are looking out of your eyes from deep within them, with a soft unfocused gaze. Imagine spaciousness inside your mouth.

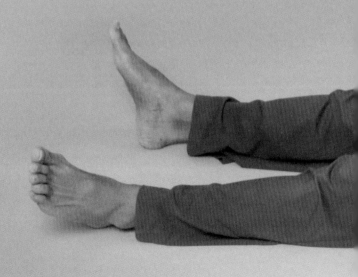

7. Then bring your attention to your chest: imagine the inner surface of your rib cage, its whole circumference becoming more open, wider and deeper. Be sure you are just imagining it and not trying to increase its volume by actually doing something.

8. Now bring your attention to the abdomen: allow this fluid-filled area to settle and sink. Let the abdominal muscles soften and sense a deepening behind the navel. Finally, take a few deeper breaths and really let the exhalation go, like a deep relaxing sigh.

9. To deepen the practice further, try to bring your awareness to the feeling of your body breathing. Try to distinguish the difference between watching your breath and sensing your breath. Whenever possible, come back to sensing rather than watching the breath.

SENSE OF ENQUIRY

There seem to be three main ways the mind wanders.

- Firstly, it can flit from idea to idea, thought to thought, like an idle daydream. This is almost always pleasant and linked to a creative mind. If your mind does this, simply allow it.

- Secondly, it can start planning, doing mental shopping or making lists of things to do. In this state, the mind goes into the future, and will almost certainly bring small tensions into the body with such thoughts. So if this happens, draw your awareness back to the feeling of the body breathing, so that you become immersed in sensation rather than thought.

- Finally, you may find yourself stuck in a cycle of negative rumination, going over and over a troubling thought. This is agitating and can be more difficult to quell. If this is happening, you might need some gentle distraction. You can do this by starting to control your breathing with long, slow breaths, making them smooth and steady until the thoughts start to subside.

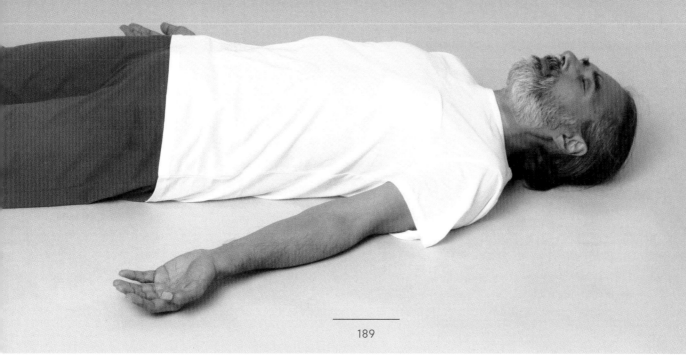

INDEX

BIBLIOGRAPHY

Butler, David, and Lorimer Moseley. *Explain Pain*. 2013. Noigroup Publications.

Cacioppo, John T. 2009. *Loneliness: Human Nature and the Need for Social Connection*. W. W. Norton & Company.

Damasio, Antonio. 2000. *The Feeling Of What Happens: Body, Emotion and the Making of Consciousness*. Vintage.

Gerhardt, Sue. 2014. *Why Love Matters: How Affection Shapes a Baby's Brain*. Routledge.

Gracovetsky, Serge. 1989. *The Spinal Engine*. Springer Verlag.

Graziano, Michael. 2009. *The Intelligent Movement Machine: An Ethological Perspective on the Primate Motor System*. OUP USA.

Keleman, Stanley. 1989. *Emotional Anatomy*. Center Press.

Mallinson, James, and Mark Singleton. 2017. *Roots of Yoga*. Penguin Classics.

O'Sullivan, Suzanne. 2016. *It's All in Your Head: Stories from the Frontline of Psychosomatic Illness*. Vintage.

Panksepp, Jaak. 2004. *Affective Neuroscience: The Foundations of Human and Animal Emotions*. Oxford University Press, USA

Sacks, Oliver. 2011. *The Man Who Mistook His Wife for a Hat*. Picador Classics.

Singleton, Mark. 2010. *Yoga Body: The Origins of Modern Posture Practice*. Oxford University Press, US Muscles Alive A.

ADDITIONAL RECOMMENDED READING

Basmajian, John, and Carlo De Luca. 1985. *Muscles Alive: Their Functions Revealed by Electromyography*. Lippincott Williams and Wilkins.

Benedetti, Fabrizio. 2011. *The Patient's Brain: The Neuroscience Behind the Doctor-Patient Relationship*. Oxford University Press USA.

Biven, Lucy, and Jaak Panksepp. 2012. *The Archaeology of Mind: Neuroevolutionary Origins of Human Emotion*. W.W. Norton & Company.

Blakeslee, Sandra and Matthew. 2009. *The Body Has a Mind of its Own: How Body Maps in Your Brain Help You Do (Almost) Everything Better*. Random House USA Inc.

Capra, Fritjof, and Pier Luigi Luísi. 2014. *The Systems View of Life: A Unifying Vision*. Cambridge University Press.

Connolly, Peter. 2014. *A Student's Guide to the History and Philosophy of Yoga*. Equinox Publishing Ltd.

Feldenkrais, Moshe. 1991. *Awareness Through Movement: Easy-to-Do Health Exercises to Improve Your Posture, Vision, Imagination, and Personal Awareness*. HarperSanFrancisco.

Feldenkrais, Moshe. 2014. *Body and Mature Behaviour*. Routledge.

Fromm, Erich. 1997. *On Being Human*. Continnuum.

Fromm, Erich. 2010. *The Art of Loving*.

Grayling, A.C. 2008. *Scepticism and the Possibility of Knowledge*. Continuum.

Hanna, Thomas. 2004. *Somatics: Reawakening the Mind's Control of Movement, Flexibility, and Health*. Da Capo Press.

Kapandaji, I. A. 2010. *The Physiology of the Joints*. Churchill Livingstone.

Kramer, Joel, and Diane Alstad. 1993. *The Guru Papers: Masks of Authoritarian Power*. North Atlantic Books, USA.

Ledoux, Joseph. 1999. *The Emotional Brain: The Mysterious Underpinnings of Emotional Life*. W&N.

Lieber, Richard. 2009. *Skeletal Muscle Structure, Function, and Plasticity*. Lippincott Williams and Wilkins.

Maté, Gabor. 2013. *In the Realm of Hungry Ghosts: Close Encounters with Addiction*. Random House Canada.

Maté, Gabor. 2012. *When The Body Says No: The Cost Of Hidden Stress*. Random House Canada.

McNeill, Alexander R. *Elastic Mechanisms in Animal Movement*. 1988. Cambridge University Press.

Pinker, Steven. 2003. *The Blank Slate: The Modern Denial of Human Nature*. Penguin Press Science.

Pfeifer, Rolf. 2006. *How the Body Shapes the Way We Think: A New View of Intelligence*. MIT Press.

Shubin, Neil. 2009. *Your Inner Fish: The Amazing Discovery of Our 375-million-year-old Ancestor*. Penguin.

Storr, Anthony. 1997. *Feet of Clay: A Study of Gurus*. HarperCollins.

Van der Kolk, Bessel. 2015. *The Body Keeps the Score: Mind, Brain and Body in the Transformation of Trauma*. Penguin.

Walsh, Geoffrey. 1992. *Muscles, Masses and Motion: The Physiology of Normality, Hypotonicity, Spasticity and Rigidity*. Mac Keith Press.